GW01032939

'The Lunatic Paupe

Glenside Hospital
Bristol
1861 – 1994

Its birth, development and demise

By
Donal F. Early
Emeritus Consultant Psychiatrist

You may break you may shatter the vase if you will
But the scent of the roses will linger around still
Thomas Moore

Conceived, created and written by Dr Donal Early

Initial layout with help of Ann Early

Edited for publication by Dr Peter Carpenter

Copyright Dr Donal Early 2003

Published by

Friends of Glenside Hospital Museum
University of the West of England Glenside Campus
Stapleton
Bristol BS16 1DD

IBSN: 0-9542458-2-2

Foreword

Dr. Donal Early was born in Ireland in 1917. He was educated at Clongoes Wood College, County Kildare and at the College of Surgeons in Dublin. He qualified in 1941 with L.R.C.P.&S.I. He later obtained a D.P.H and D.P.M from Dublin.

He moved to England in 1944 joining the staff of the Bristol Mental Hospital. This story is told in the book.

He is a foundation member of the Royal College of Psychiatrists and was for many years W.H.O. adviser in Rehabilitation.

This book was written over many years. Dr Early suffered a stroke in 2001 leaving him with aphasia. The chapter on *The Glensider* was completed after the stroke.

Ann Early

Contents

List of Illustrations

Colour Plates   *inserted between pages 42 & 43*

Paintings by Stanley Spencer at Sandham Memorial Chapel, Burghclere

Poem

He sits and sits and sits all day;
People marry: go Holiday: work, even play;
People feel happy: write books, read books, books many;
People have visitors, he doesn't want any.

   He just sits.

A sweet child, my son, and happy at school,
Erstwhile a Student, keen as a rule;
He could run, he could swim, he could ski;
Why can't he feel free?

   He just sits.

Not sunk in despair, though at 40 life's spent
In a Hospital arm-chair, grimly content;
In a void he can't fill;
No-one's to blame he is mentally ill.

   He just sits.

Why should he want _me_? Why care for _me_?
I am the culprit in his eyes I see;
I freely forgave one aggressive attack.
Now I should love to receive him back.

   He just sits.

I grieved for my loss. I prayed for my son.
One day I found that my faith had won.
Came my 80th Birthday, came joy at last;
I tore open the envelope keenly and fast……………….

  Perhaps he had risen from sitting?

Hand-writing well-known from old days gone by.
A beautiful Card and chosen with care; I couldn't but cry.
Remembrance and love and good wishes he sends.
How are you? He asks; our love never ends.

So for once, just for me, he climbed out of his chair;
Praise God I'm forgiven, with love that we share.
Oh! Could he recover, feel happy again?
That the burden of years had not all been in vain.

By a Founder-Member of the National Schizophrenic Fellowship.
Christmas 1987.

Preface

Attempts to record the history of individual mental hospitals have varied greatly being usually restricted by financial restraints and coloured by the experiences of individual authors. Some like the Short History of Rubery Hill which covers 100 years of service to Birmingham in a 16 page essay cannot be compared with the affluent 150 year History of St Andrew's Hospital Northampton, co-edited by a professional journalist. There are many admirable soft back booklets with high standard of research and composition like those which relate the story of De La Pole Hospital, of the Old Hull Borough Asylum, of Stanley Royd, of St Mathew's, Burntwood all of which differ in approach from David Clarke's personally told story of Fulbourn Hospital, Cambridge, as much as from the Dark Awakening, Dr C J Andrews tribute to St Lawrence's Hospital, Bodmin – dedicated "to the staff of Cornwall Lunatic Asylum and Cornwall Mental Hospital, who for one hundred and thirty years held the line until public opinion awoke and the darkness was dispelled."

All the histories, short or long, attempt something of patient conditions and to record the poorly requited service of Asylum and of Mental Hospital workers, a group of men and women whose near-impossible problems have rarely been sympathetically perceived. In 1961 on the occasion of the centenary of the now defunct Glenside Hospital,[1] J. L. (Laurie) Davis, the last Clerk and Steward of Bristol Mental Hospital and the first Secretary of its Hospital Management Committee put together a roneo-duplicated history of the hospital. He had little or no encouragement and no financial backing. He gathered together abstracts from the annual reports of the Visiting Committee, the Hospital Management Committee (H.M.C.), the Commissioners in Lunacy and of the Board of Control, the Medical Superintendent and the hospital Chaplain. The result is an account of hospital activities seen through the eyes of a fair-minded trusted administrator with some of the day-to-day hospital atmosphere occasionally breaking through. He seldom related any of the many difficulties with which he had to contend.[2]

There can rarely have been a more dedicated team than the staff of Glenside in the post-war years. Up to 1972/73, they maintained an incomparable morale under conditions which at times could have overwhelmed them. The condition of Fishponds was underprivileged *vis a vis* Barrow Hospital which functioned under the same Hospital Management Committee and which will be recurrently referred to throughout our story. Lest it be thought that there is an element of whingeing in this, a brief reference to the comparative costs of maintenance will clearly indicate the nub of the problem. On 19th September, Mr Forbes the hospital treasurer, reported to the Finance Committee that the difference between the costs of Fishponds and Barrow "is so marked that it has been highlighted by the Regional Board Treasurer who has submitted a statement to the Board's Finance Committee showing the excess expenditure for the year 1964/65 compared with the national average for Barrow and Fishponds amounted to £103,225.00 and as Glenside was below the national average, the excess must be attributed to Barrow Hospital." That year the national average figure was £11-05-11d [£11.30p]. Barrow Hospital was £18-10-01d [£18.50p]. Again in 1966/67 Glenside cost £12-15-05d [£12.77p]. Barrow £21-14-02d [£21.74p]. The Treasurer again commented on the disparity and weakly suggested that "it may be possible by constant comparison and if necessary by ad hoc investigations to suggest economies." But things did not change.

The dissolution of the mental hospitals makes it important that their past should be recorded. Glenside Hospital, is already a fading memory. Happily the buildings being listed could not be sold for commercial development. The rape of the main estate has thus been avoided, except for 2½ acres on the opposite side of the main road, Blackberry Hill, which was sold for £2,500,000 for a housing development.

---

[1] The name Glenside was the correct name after 1959 but the old name – Fishponds, was frequently used after this.
[2] His work has been reprinted by the Glenside Hospital Museum.

After the Great Displacement of its patients the hospital first became the Avon College of Health, later the Avon and Gloucester College of Health and in March 1996 the Faculty of Health and Social Care of the University of the West of England.

The story which I shall relate will try to trace the establishment of the Bristol Borough Lunatic Asylum in 1861, its rapid early enlargement and its development through decades of relentless change to closure in 1994.

The story will unavoidably be skewed by my personal experiences, which began on May 4th 1944 immediately after the appointment of Robert Hemphill as Medical Superintendent. Unlike David Clarke I started in the most junior medical position without the benefits of his considerable experience and authority.

I had completed a mere 6 months as a Clinical Clerk in Grangegoram Mental Hospital, Dublin which included 2 months locum Assistant Medical Officer (A.M.O.). My theoretical interest in Psychiatry had been blunted by the apparent hopelessness of the condition of patients who had little hope of improvement, recovery or discharge, crowded together in a hospital, which dated from 1815 with no plans for change. Status as a Clinical Clerk precluded any but the slightest contribution to the improvement of patient welfare. There were 5 clinical doctors for 3000 plus patients. Little wonder that the professional attitude of the time was one of laissez-faire. Dr E.A. Waldron who was leaving his job as Assistant Medical Officer at Fishponds to join the R.A.F. recommended me to the Bristol Mental Hospital, Fishponds. This was followed by an invitation from Dr Robert Hemphill to join the staff. I arrived in Bristol at 2am on May 4th 1944 and started work on the same day.

For more than 35 years I worked daily with the patients and staff of Fishponds Hospital. They were an unforgettable bunch. Of course, some were more memorable than others but they all deserved better than they received. This poor hard-begotten mouse of a book belongs to them. I acknowledge my debit to them.

Sarah Cook, Custodian of the Stanley Spencer Memorial Chapel at Burghclere, where so much lingers of old Fishponds helped me to appreciate the glimpses there of the Beaufort War Hospital. My secretary Gill Wadsworth put up with me through periods of near despair, my friend Ken Harris helped to illuminate pictorially my dull script. John Bird, Reader in Psychology in the Faculty of Economies and Social Sciences in the University of the West of England, lent me a good story of Dr Thompson culled from his unpublished book "Madness, Crime and Politics." My grateful thanks to them but to none more so than to my wife who can never be requited for her knowledge, patience and endurance which have supported me in this as in all aspects of our lives together.

Fifty-five years of association with Glenside Hospital, 35 as a practising psychiatrist have seen the metamorphosis of a closed to an open hospital, to closure. Personal association with many of the changes has not guaranteed an awareness of diverse activities which were part of hospital life throughout the years. To distil the information gleaned from many sources during and after my association with the hospital and to weave it into a coherent story became increasingly difficult with every fresh enquiry. Closeness to the task makes it impossible to maintain the distance and detachment necessary for the production an unbiased narrative. Perhaps the task should have been undertaken by someone else, but it wasn't. I ask indulgence when the facts are unduly coloured by personal experience and prejudice.

Donal Early

St. Peter's Hospital, Bristol 1698

There are many claims to have been the first-established hospital for the treatment and care of the mentally ill. The City of Valencia has no doubt that the sermon of Padre Juan Joffre on February 24th 1409 led to the foundation of the world's first hospital specifically for the care and treatment of the mentally ill. On March 15th 1410 Lorenzo Salom with 9 other merchants of Valencia were granted a decree by King Martin el Humano to found the Spital de Ignocents, Folls e Orats, which continued into the 20th century as the Sanatorio Psiquiatrico Provincial del Padre Joffre.

Almost 300 years later in 1695 John Carey, a Bristol merchant published "An Essay on the State of England in Relation to its Trade, its poor and its Taxes for carrying on the present War against France." This was printed and issued by W. Bonny, Bristol, November 1695, the first book to be issued from a Bristol printing press. The following year Carey issued from the same press, a folio sheet entitled "Proposals for the better Maintaining and Imploying the Poor of the City of Bristol Humbly referred to the consideration of the Mayor." The proposals were incorporated in the Bristol Poor Act 1696 which anticipated Gilberts Act of 1782 and established a new system of poor law administration in Bristol, "the prototype of the work house" which later became general throughout the country. The new scheme led to the combination of all 18 parishes of the city in one area, with one building in which the destitute and the homeless poor would be maintained at one uniform rate, levied in each parish, carried to a common fund to meet the cost of relief. In this institution the able-bodied would be compelled to work, the infirm would be well cared for, the young would be adequately trained, expenditure would be saved and litigation between parishes would disappear. It also undertook to admit pauper lunatics, a unique step forward, rendered even more enlightened by the guiding principles, which were laid down, that they should receive treatment and not punishment, that they be provided with living conditions adapted to their needs, that their wards be floored with planks and adequately covered with straw and that chains were not to be used.[1]

The Poor Act established a Board of Guardians, consisting of a Governor, Deputy Governor, Assistants and Guardians of the Poor which first met in St George's Chapel the Guildhall on 19th of May 1696. The Workhouse called Whitehall adjoining the Bridewell was selected and furnished at an outlay of £260 and soon 100 girls were being trained as carders and spinners and being taught to read. The room was insufficient and in December 1697 it was decided, to buy for £800, the Old Sugar House currently occupied by the Mint. There was difficulty prising out the officer in charge, so that the purchase was not completed until 7th June 1698, in which year it was opened as St Peter's Hospital. Measures were taken to train 110 boys to weave. The porter's wife was ordered to teach them to read and due provision was made for disciplinary apparatus including a pair of stocks, a whipping post and a place of confinement styled "Purgatory", fitted with chains and fetter locks.

The first meeting of the Corporation of the Poor was held on 20th October 1698. In 1865 part of the premises were disposed of "reserving only the interesting and picturesque mansion for the Board and financial offices, all happily well-preserved and cared for by its Poor Law Owners." This happy state was shattered in March 1940 when the building and its contents were destroyed by enemy bombing.

Initially the treatment of lunatics in St Peter's was enlightened. A medical consultant was appointed at the meeting of the Board in December 1697: "It being represented to this court by Mr Edward Hackett and Mr James Millard that Dr Thomas Dover hath offered himself to be Phisitian to the new Workhouse gratis, this Court doth accept him as such and do order

---

[1] J. J. Simpson 'St Peters' Hospital Bristol.' *Bristol Archaeological Notes XVI* 1924–1929 Vol XLVII pp193-226.

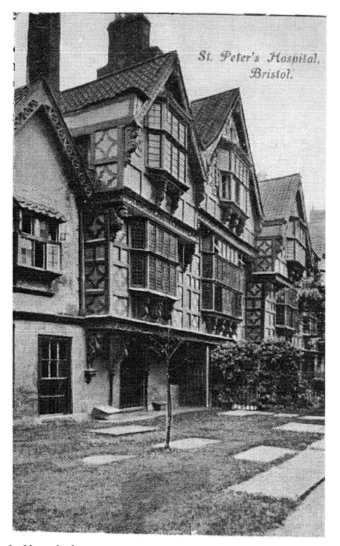

Figure 1 St Peter's Hospital

that the said Mr Hackett and Mr Millard do give him notice thereof and also that this Court do thank him for ye same." Dr Dover thus became the first doctor appointed to a lunatic ward. He was a grandson of Robert Dover who instituted the 'Commonwealth Olimpick Games' on Dover Hill, Weston–sub–Edge, Gloucester. He was a medical practitioner in Bristol from 1696 to 1708. He then became part-owner and second in command of the Duke privateer which with its sister ship the Duchess circumnavigated the world in 1708 under Captain Woodes Rogers. He was in charge of the landing party from the Duke who rescued Alexander Selkirk (Robinson Crusoe) from the island of Juan Fernandez where he had spent 4 ½ years.

By 1700 there were about 300 persons under the care of the Guardians. In 1712 St Peter's was enlarged and reconstructed by Robert Ashworth. At this time it was described as the prototype of workhouses. In the early years the lunatic ward conditions appear to have been good but having made these pioneering strides, Bristol ran out of steam. As the 18th century passed, conditions grew progressively worse although no criticism is presented in Matthew's New History of Bristol 1793-4 (A Complete Guide and Bristol Directory for the year 1793-4). Where St Peter's is placed first amongst the "Hospitals, Almshouses and charitable institutes (which) are so numerous that we must content ourselves with little more than announcing them. St Peter's Hospital in St Peter's Street is the general hospital for the poor of the whole city including superannuated persons, orphans, and ideots; it has a ward for lunatics. Vagrants and beggars are taken up and sent hither. The building is ancient and very spacious, and was the mansion of Thomas Norton Esq. M.P. for Bristol in 1399; afterwards, the Mint for the coinage of money, which is now its most general title and in the

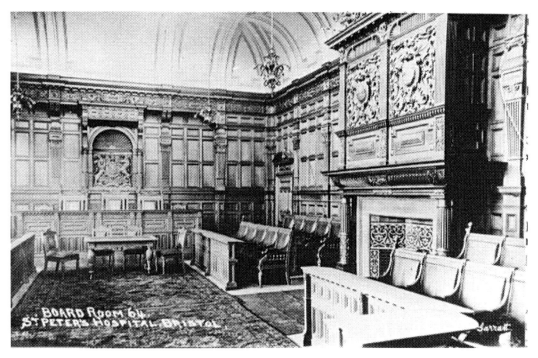

Figure 2 The Boardroom at St Peter's Hospital

8th of William 3rd erected into the City Hospital with a governor, deputy, treasurer, guardians, physitian, apothecary, chaplain and other officers. It is supported by an annual assesment on the parishes of Bristol."

This bland description may have been valid at the time but it did not fit for long. Conditions, worsened in the 19th century. In 1827 there were three lunatic wards. Ward 14 (Bedlam, female) Ward 16 (Upper Bedlam, female) and Ward 20 (Bedlam male). In 1839 "paupers were mixed with lunatics, whether imbecile or violent with little or no protection" and "the present sleeping room for the lunatics was more likely to engender disease than to cure it, for a more melancholy department the writer has never seen." (John Latimer. The Annals of Bristol in the Nineteenth Century W&F Morgan Clare Street, Bristol 1887).

In 1830, John Latimer, Editor of the *Bristol Mercury* describes vividly the deterioration, which had overtaken conditions in St Peter's. Trade was depressed during the following two years "causing members of the labouring classes to fall into pauperism. As the City Workhouse, St Peter's Hospital had even before the distress, been full to repletion, the increased demand for relief plunged the Corporation of the Poor into extreme embarrassment." The Armoury or 'Ordinance Barracks', Stapleton Road, was bought for £3,100.00 for the reception of pauper lunatics. This "was, however, first postponed and then abandoned, it being deemed inadvisable to impose further taxation whilst the ratepayers were groaning under the burdens inflicted upon them by events about to be narrated." A labourer out of work with a wife and 5 children got 10s1d (50.5p) per week outdoor relief – stone-breaking 8 hours per day for 4 days. An agricultural labourer's wage was only 9s (45p) per week for more than double the quantity of work. Thus "demand for pauper relief became daily more formidable." Able–bodied paupers were ordered by guardians to work 5 days per week, 10½ hours daily, for an additional sum of 4d weekly. But "they rose in revolt when the announcement was made and for a time St Peter's Hospital was in great peril. The mayor and aldermen however acted with great promptitude and firmness. The Riot Act was read, a body of troops was brought to the spot and some of the ringleaders were sent to prison. The energy of the magistrates put an end to the disturbance and the paupers submitted to the new scale. The pressures on St Peter's Hospital, continued and the building, gorged with 600 inmates became most unhealthy, as well as a sink of moral contamination. According to an authentic contemporary statement, 58 girls slept in 10 beds and between 70 or 80 boys in 17 beds.

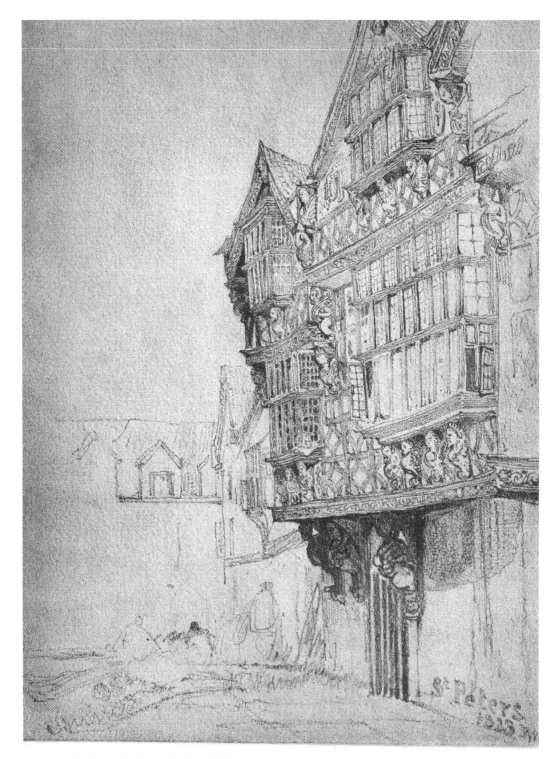

Figure 3 St Peter's Hospital in 1823

The Guardians found themselves compelled to set about long needed reforms and in 1833 another disused building belonging to the Government, the former   French Prison at Stapleton was hired from the Admiralty at a rent of £80 a year, put in repair and fitted up for a considerable number of paupers. The experiment proved satisfactory and the building in 1837 was purchased for £3,000.00.

After nearly 150 years, the glory of the pioneering lunatic treatment was gravely tarnished. In 1840, the lunatics in St Peter's were confined in pens 7ft x 3ft 2ins for men and 6ft x 3ft for women. In 1841 the Justices recommended straps instead of handcuffs and irons and they objected to women wearing masks or muzzles "such as are put on dogs." They

4

recommended that lunatics be sent to Dr Ducks asylum at Rudgeway or to Dr Bompas' (private) asylum at Fishponds, until suitable accommodation was secured.

The population of Bristol was expanding rapidly. The conditions in St Peter's could scarcely have been worse. In 1844 the Lunacy Commissioners inspected all the mad houses and asylums in the country and expressed "almost unqualified censure" on 32 existing institutions. They described St Peter's unequivocally as "totally unfit for an asylum." They recommended that the entire body of lunatics ought to be moved to more spacious premises and to more healthy and airy situation.

> The part of the Bristol Workhouse called St. Peter's Hospital, set apart for the Pauper Lunatics of the city, is without any day-room, eating-room, or kitchen, for the Females, distinct from their sleeping apartments; and the only place in which they (40 in number) can take exercise is a small passage or paved yard at one end of the Hospital. It is part of the road for carts to the Workhouse, and measures about 37 feet by 18, and is, from its pavement and extent utterly unfit for an airing-ground. The accommodations for the men are somewhat better, but they have only part of a paved yard, very little larger that that appropriated to the Females. ... There are small wooden closets, or Pens, for confining the violent and refractory Patients. Those for the men were 7 feet long by 3 feet 3 inches broad, and about 9 feet high, and were warmed by pipes, and had a hole in the door, and also a hole in the ceiling for ventilation. The Pens for the Women were smaller and were not warmed, and were ill ventilated. The walls of each were of wood, but were not padded. Formerly, Patients were occasionally kept in those Pens during both day and night, but the Pens are now very rarely used ... In addition to the jacket and leg-locks, a sort of open mask of leather passing round the face, and also round the forehead to the back of the head, and fastened by leather straps, was at one time placed over the heads of such Patients as were in the habit of biting; but this mask (as the Commissioners understand) has been for some time discontinued.[1]

Since 1809 the Local Authorities had a duty to provide accommodation for pauper lunatics. In 1845 the Lunatics Act made this a mandatory duty. The City fathers vacillated whilst conditions in St Peters deteriorated. Sixteen long years more were to pass before Bristol's Asylum was built.

In their 1847 report the Commissioners in Lunacy reported that 27 of the 64 patients admitted to St. Peters in the previous 13 months had died. They considered that "this mortality appears considerable." They recorded the failure of their repeated attempts to persuade the Guardians to provide suitable accommodation and concluded that "the wards and yards at present set aside for the Insane Poor of Bristol are totally unfit for the purpose" that "the present arrangement is utterly discreditable and unless the Corporation takes measures for its amendment, the condition of the Insane Poor of Bristol will require the intervention of some higher authority." In September 1849 the Council informed the Secretary of State that they had done all that they could for the improvement of conditions in St Peters and since Bristol already had accommodation for pauper lunatics they (the Commissioners) had no power to force the provision of an alternative building. They requested the Secretary of State to suspend his compulsory powers. In October 1853 a new Secretary of State, Palmerston, brought the matter up again. The Mayor expressed surprise explaining that Bristol did have an asylum. But by now even the local press had become highly critical. The *Bristol Mirror and General Advertizer* reported the conclusions of a Committee appointed by the Board of Guardians that the position of St Peters in the centre of the City rendered it "unfit and inadequate for a County Asylum... The dangerous and harmless, curable and incurable, dirty and clean, noisy and quiet are all associated together in one common room... the County Lunatic Asylum should be entirely independent of the workhouse..."

Year by year criticism mounted. The mentally ill of other counties benefited from the 1845 Act, but not Bristol. Continuing evasion of this responsibility by the Corporation led to

---

[1] 1844 Report of the Metropolitan Commissioners in Lunacy.

increasing insistence by the Home Office. A prolonged confrontation ensued. Order after order from the Home Office was ignored. In November 1854 deferment was again requested by the Corporation "so as to avoid heavy expenditure by the ratepayers, when already they are spending heavily on sewage and other sanitary measures under the Public Health Act." The Under Secretary of State replied that Lord Palmerston regretted that the reasons for delay were "not sufficient for continuance of so great a practical evil" and turned up the heat by issuing a further Order on December 23rd 1854.

The City still thought to evade its statutory duty but throughout January/February 1855, the Council and the Corporation of the Poor were at loggerheads. The Council favoured the transfer of paupers to Stapleton Workhouse with St Peters being given over for the exclusive use of lunatics, whilst the Corporation of the Poor held the opposite view, adding that lunatics "do not require a fine place to reside in." In May the two bodies agreed to a committee of 14, seven members from each "to endeavour to postpone the building of a new lunatic asylum."

By September nothing had happened and the Corporation received another order from the Home Secretary which the Mayor referred to as "that tremendous evil which overhangs the City." The following week, the Joint Committee met. It was admitted that the St Peter's wards for lunatics were inadequate but it was argued that city people being accustomed to urban confinement required different facilities than country people and that, therefore, St Peters could be up-graded to the standards necessary for city lunatics and that this "would obviate the necessity of offering benefits for a few unfortunate objects which would not be duly appreciated." One further suggestion that accommodation be sought with a neighbouring asylum was rejected but no agreement was possible during the following three months. The local newspapers (*Bristol Gazette, Bristol Mirror and General Advertizer, Bristol Mercury*). reported an increasing volume of opposition to the proposition to build. This was orchestrated by the Mayor and became increasingly raucous. By October the *Bristol Gazette* described building an asylum as "lunacy itself" and urged acceptance by the Minister of an offer of beds in Stapleton workhouse with 4½ acres of land attached. The *Gazette* agreed that the Secretary of State had power to compel compliance with his orders and that everything should be done which was necessary for the afflicted inmates but averred that "to take a pauper simply because he is mad and to place him in a palace with pleasure grounds, ornamental water etc., is nothing short of philanthropy gone mad." The *Mirror* said:

> We certainly admire the pertinacity with which the Guardians have held at arms length the Commissioners in Lunacy. Since 1843 these gentlemen have been continually reporting on the utter worthlessness of St Peters Hospital... and here we are in the year 1855 and you may still hear the melancholy cry of these poor creatures as they look out upon the Avon through the strongly barred windows. The Home Secretary is becoming peremptory and the Commissioners inexorable. Indeed, unless some settlement of the question is speedily come to, we shall have our worthy Mayor seized in his bed together with all the Town Council and incarcerated for contempt of Court, for such is the punishment that Municipal Authorities are liable to who defy the mandates of Government... The only alternative to seeing our whole Corporation, Mayor and all sent off to prison is to saddle ourselves with a debt varying from £50,000 to £175,000, as fate and the architect might will it.... We are asked to provide Pauper Lunatics with a palace which will cost us from £200 to £700 per idiot or madman. It must be a positive pleasure, to be out of ones mind in the present day. But we must take care that we are not reducing sound minds to a similar state of insanity... We are not at all surprised to find the citizens assembling in their wards to escape this fresh impost and all that will entail hereafter. If the Commissioners in Lunacy were answerable to the citizens in any way, they could perhaps be more moderate in their ideas."[1]

The paper commented that the Commissioners would be too proud to accept a renovation of St Peters or an expansion of the workhouse to meet their requirements at a third of the cost

---

[1] *Bristol Mirror* leader on October 10th 1855

of their plan and it recommended that a deputation visit Lord Palmerston to plead the City's case "for not commencing at once the Lunatic Pauper Palace."

Public meetings were addressed by the Mayor. To the parishes of St James & St Paul he said "Why! your lunatic asylums are royal palaces surrounded by princely domains." He described the Order of the Secretary of State as an awful missile suspended like the sword of Damocles by a single hair over the heads of the Citizens of Bristol. In spite of his demagogy he knew that conditions had to change. This densely crowded and later similar meetings were persuaded by him to propose that Stapleton workhouse should be developed for the use of the pauper lunatics. The Town Council recommended accordingly but no acceptable compromise could be reached with the Poor Law Commissioners who remained in favour of allocating St Peter's for the sole use of lunatics. The only agreement possible was that the Home Office should not insist upon palaces being built for lunatics "not one of which could appreciate them" according to the *Bristol Mercury* on October 27th 1855.

The *Mirror* still veered toward compromise. Sebastapol having fallen on 8th September, it recommended that St Peter's continue to provide accommodation until the end of the war and then perhaps a new asylum might be the best option. It added "It is all very well to grow sentimental over pauper lunatics [but] as the Mayor has very shrewdly said there is a tendency to lavish a mawkish sensibility on lunatics, prisoners etc. but an almost complete indifference to the struggle of that class of the population which is the most numerous in the land – the small taxpayer."

On December 27th 1855 the Council resolved to develop the Stapleton site and sent a deputation to the Poor Law Commissioners to procure their consent to the appropriation of Stapleton Workhouse for the purpose of an asylum. There was no agreement. In April 1856 the Poor Law Commissioners refused permission for the sale of part of Stapleton for an asylum but in any case this was no longer an option. The Lunacy Commissioners would not again turn a blind eye. The political power of the Centre was overwhelming. The hospital had to be built by agreement or by compulsory order. Minor bickering continued throughout the coming months but a decision to build was taken, however reluctantly. The Council conceded defeat in May 1856 and wrote to the Commissioners who in turn sent to them a Paper of Suggestions for the building of the Asylum stressing the need for economy.

In July 1856 the City Council considered 8 possible sites and in March 1857, Fishponds was approved. J.R. Lysaght, a local architect of Imperial Chambers, Bristol was commissioned to produce plans for an asylum to be built on a site next to Stapleton workhouse. Work began tardily in 1858 and proceeded slowly. When the first patients were transferred from St Peters to Fishponds in March 1861, the building work was still incomplete.

Bristol Lunatic Asylum: The First Decade

Doctor Henry Oxley Stephens, the first Medical Superintendent of the Fishponds Asylum had previously been the Superintendent of St Peters Hospital. His first annual report was generally congratulatory and understanding of the Visiting Committees problems, although he clearly stated that there could be no doubt that the conditions in St Peters were so poor, "that another asylum was imperatively required." He must of course have been aware that his Chairman William Herepath was opposed to the building of a new asylum, he having been in favour of assigning St Peters Hospital to the exclusive use of the mentally ill. He was Chairman of the Asylum Committee of Visitors for the first two years. His first report was almost completely designed to assure his fellow Councillors that he and his Committee would safeguard the financial interests of the ratepayers.

It had been estimated that 120 patients would be transferred from St Peter's to the new asylum and it was realised that the expenditure per patient in St Peter's would not be sufficient for the new hospital. Allowing for this number of patients being attended by 27 servants @ £26 per annum there would be a short fall of £342 at the years end. This necessitated an increase in the charge to City Parishes from 10/- [50p] to 12/- [60p] per week and to Parishes outside the City 14/- [70p] per week from 12/-. The small excess of income that this brought, did not cover the costs entailed by the incomplete arrangements when the asylum was opened and by the smaller than anticipated number of patients transferred. It was therefore necessary to borrow £500. Although the number of patients at the year's end was 160, the asylum had not become self-supporting and the debt was not being reduced. Mr Herepath said that when three months income in advance was in-hand, the weekly charge would be reduced and that "all parties have in view only one objective, which is to economise the public funds as much as possible." By the end of year two, when the number of patients had reached 180, the Chairman pointed out that grave financial embarrassment was caused by the heavy expenses attending the management of a small asylum designed for 200 patients. "The same amount of attendance and general management which is necessary for 180 patients will suffice for 250", he said and added that in Wells and in Gloucester Asylums the population varied between 500 and 600 "with general staff nearly the same as ours."

The seeds of overcrowding were thus sown in the second year of the hospital's existence. Overcrowding progressed much more rapidly than was anticipated. This socially and medically unhappy state, which was due to the accumulation of incurable patients, was greeted with satisfaction by the Chairman who announced that the charge for City Patients would soon be reduced. He repeated financial assurances which could hardly have been more uncompromising but having noted the additional buildings which had been provided, strong-rooms for refractory patients, a bakery, a piggery, a smithy, he still wished to assure

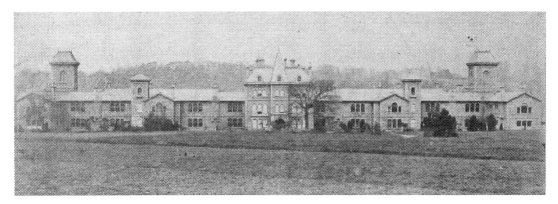

Figure 4 The Asylum as first built

the citizens that the asylum has been the cheapest in the Kingdom and that the system of management evolved by the Visitors "will compensate the ratepayers for the heavy burdens that so large and expensive an asylum have necessarily entailed upon them." He remained predominantly concerned with the soundness of the financial arrangements of his committee. He repeated the view that the hospital was too small to be financially self-supporting and continued to be envious of the larger neighbouring hospitals in Wells and in Gloucester. He bemoaned the costly method of conducting Lunatic Asylums which made the expenses per head considerably greater than that of paupers in the workhouse.

A liberal regime which was established, "no mechanical restraint, not a straight waistcoat on the premises", strained his tolerance and he complained of damage "of considerable magnitude" done to clothing by destructive patients which "in one or more cases amounted to a sum which if your Committee were to state it, would be deemed incredible." Whilst not overtly objecting to the fact that mechanical restraint had not been employed in the asylum, he had his doubts about the wisdom of this, although "it is the theory of the present day and the Commissioners in Lunacy require that mechanical restraint shall not be resorted to." On the other hand he recorded with approbation that much help had been given to the hospital by patients most of whom were orderly, helpful and well conducted. They helped with housework. All the hospital clothing and shoes were made on the premises and the piggeries made a handsome profit but whilst pleased with these aspects of activity, he considered that employment should not only be productive of profit but should contribute to the ultimate recovery of patients.

He ended his second and last report as he began, by unfavourably comparing the maintenance rate of the asylum with that of its bigger neighbours and adjured his successor to use his utmost endeavours to assist in getting costs down. In 1863 he resigned the Chair in favour of Mr Frederick Terrill, by which time the number of in-patients had risen to 199 and an extension of accommodation was proposed.

The medical appreciation of the new asylum in the annual reports was almost unbridled. There can be no doubting the genuine happiness of Dr Stephens in observing the effect of the "light airy and cheerful residence" which greeted his patients on transfer from St Peters. On February 27th 1861 "a boon to suffering humanity" was delivered when 50 men from St Peters Hospital were transferred. Six days later 63 women joined them. In spite of his joy he could not refrain from commenting on the past political difficulties. He lamented "that a great and opulent city ...(with) magnificent infirmaries and hospitals for the relief of the sick poor, asylums for deserted orphans, and alms houses for repose of the aged, should have remained so long destitute of any place at all for the suitable reception and treatment of persons afflicted with mental maladies, a class of sufferers who make the strongest appeal to our commiseration."

He referred to the ill-arranged and deficient accommodation of St Peters with its jail-like and depressing appearance, overcrowded conditions and lack of exercising and airing grounds. He described how almost every patient from St Peters improved physically and mentally and how patients whose behaviour was previously perverse, intractable, destructive and dirty, became docile, orderly, clean and fittingly employed.

The Commissioners in Lunacy who visited the asylum on 23rd March 1861, less than three weeks after the hospital opened, said that they "could hardly recognise the patients before them as the same company they had been accustomed to seeing in St Peters Hospital."

Dr Stephens' regime was liberal. He stressed the importance of employment, the intention of which was to benefit the patients more than to provide gain for the hospital. He disapproved of mechanical restraint which was not employed nor was the straight waistcoat.

He believed in the curative value of retirement and quiet contemplation in solitude; he allowed enforced seclusion in rare cases to prevent self-injury.

He lamented the tendency for patients to be sent to his care only when they had become intolerably disturbed or chronically sick and disabled. The authorities tended to retain patients in the workhouse, as long as possible, it being less expensive than the asylum. The medical condition of those presented, their number and the method of their admission drew vigorous medical criticism year after year. He complained that they were very often in a disease-ridden and exhausted state. In the euphoria of the early days, he thought "that the opprobrium of an augmented mortuary list, if it be an opprobrium (should) be cheerfully borne." As the cure rate remained stubbornly low and as the beds became full, his tolerance waned and he became increasingly dissatisfied by the choice of patients for admission and by the methods of making these decisions. He criticised the Lunacy Acts Amendments Act of 1862 which required the Relieving Officer to report to a Justice of the Peace any pauper within his parish who seemed to be of unsound mind and he chided the Relieving Officers for avoiding further responsibility by obtaining a warrant for reception into the District Asylum thereby converting it into an infirmary for the sick and the dying. His grievances went unheard. Each year brought a lesser number of treatable patients. The year of 1863 was worse than 1862: eighteen epileptics were admitted and twenty patients with the mental and corporeal decay of age and intemperance, pulmonary diseases and the exhaustion of approaching dissolution. Most were incredibly filthy, some suffered from contagious diseases, consumption, old age, scrofula (glandular swelling and a tendency to consumption), chronic cerebral disease, cancer, old injuries to the head. Admission of these patients saved the Poor Law considerable amounts of money and the Asylum had no option but to admit them. With the current lunacy law whereby anyone certified appropriately had to be admitted, there was no way of avoiding an accumulation of incurable patients. However this same problem was being repeated all over the country.

The provisions of the Lunacy Amendment Act 1862 which allowed transfer of quiet patients from the asylum to the Union House gave no relief because in the Imbecile Wards of the Union these inmates soon became unmanageable again and had to be re-admitted. This great medico-administrative enigma continued to feed the remorseless increase in bed numbers. By 1866, there were up to 225 patients in the Fishponds Asylum. Patients with chronic illness continued to accumulate into conditions of hopeless institutionalism, a situation, which continued until social changes and advances in medical treatment began to reverse the trend in the nineteen-fifties.

Extensive statistical tables and comments on the main medical problems were included in each annual superintendent's report. In the first year Dr Stephens spoke of his views on the aetiology of mental illness. He disagreed with the strong impression that Asylums were tenanted by people with vices, especially drunkenness or that patients were the authors of their calamitous condition. He considered mental illness to be induced "by a variety of troubles and misfortunes, mental, moral and physical to which all are liable."

He found many clinical problems puzzling and often disturbing and he became increasingly pessimistic. Most of the patients were incurable like the man who was admitted from the Bristol Infirmary and "died of visceral disease the consequence of Australia fever" soon after admission. In 1861 he described 2 cases of General Paralysis of the Insane (GPI) (a condition not then known to be of syphilitic origin) in women which "was supposed to be confined to the male but is now frequently a cause of death in women." In a later report he recorded 3 patients who died "of that mysterious and as yet incompletely understood disease, general paralysis of the insane a condition from which it is generally assumed none recover." Year by year an estimate was made of the number of patients who were thought to be recoverable, usually half or less of those admitted. The ordinary sources of asylum mortality continued to be senile decay, phthisis [Tuberculosis], general paralysis and cerebral disorganisation of long standing associated with epilepsy or paralysis. Diseases associated with overcrowding continued, tuberculosis and Autumn diarrhoea were prevalent and occasionally fatal. There was cholera in the City in 1869.

He often discussed epilepsy, one of the most serious medical and management problems of the age. About 15% of the asylum patients and a high proportion of admissions suffered from epilepsy. In 1862 he discussed its incidence as being associated with every form and grade of mental alienation and therefore difficult to treat, "particularly in view of its peculiar proneness to vicious habits and propensities which render supervision difficult." He expressed little hope or expectation that a specific remedy would be discovered for this intractable disease especially "remembering the eulogiums formerly passed on digitalis,[1] oil of turpentine[2]" and nitrate of silver,[3] and lately on the cotyledon umbilicus[4] and phosphorus."[5] He tried a tincture of sambul root as recommended by Dr Boyd of Somerset Asylum but found it to be ineffective. He conducted a trial in six selected cases of epilepsy, two males and four females of concentrated juice of the Galium Mollage[6] or heath-bed straw, a common Bristol plant used in many of the hospitals in the South of France and "asserted to be a specific for the insane." There was no appreciable effect in five whilst one male patient had the frequency of fits reduced. He concluded "that it is scarcely probable that any active principle will be found in the section of Rubiacial to which Galium Mollage belongs." He did report the "apparent cure" of a female patient, epileptic since childhood who had been free from fits for 18 months. The re-establishment of general health steadily persevered in, led to marked improvement with decrease in the frequency and severity of paroxysms, progressive gain in coherence and improvement in temper tantrums.

In one of his reports, Dr Stephens expressed the opinion that lunatics confined in asylums are liable to become phthisical although surrounded by hygienic conditions unfavourable to the generation of tuberculosis, a good and liberal diet, warm clothing and spacious accommodation. "The explanation of this fact is that Lunatics are rendered prone to consumption not by the mental disease and confinement in an asylum as its consequence but because of the stromous diathesis which prevails among the insane and is the constitutional cause or common source of both maniacal and consumptive affections."

One of the main problems with which he had to contend was the water supply. In 1861 he confidently predicted that there would be no deficiency of water in the future which view he again expressed 6 years later referring to the abundance of water in the north side of the valley of the Frome where copious supplies were available. In the early days of the hospital the Commissioners also averred that the supply of water had never failed but in 1864 following "an almost unprecedented drought" the water supply dried up in the early summer and the expensive step had to be taken of carrying water to the hospital in carts. To combat this problem 6 acres of land were bought beside the river Frome. A tank containing 5,000 gallons of water was sunk beside the river and a pump and engine were bought to raise it to the hospital, if necessary. In spite of this in 1866 three or four patients were bathing in the same bath water. The Chairman talked of the pressing necessity for a better supply. Dr Stephens advised that there was a sufficient supply if there was great economy in

---

[1] Digitalis purpurea (Foxglove) was used in heart disease as an infusion or a tincture of digitalis leaf and the action was often uncertain.

[2] Oil of Turpentine, a distilled oil from the resin of the Scotch Fir and other species of fir, which when given internally could cause depression of the functions of the brain & spinal cord and was apt to cause strangury (painful retention of urine) and haematuria (blood in the urine).

[3] Silver nitrate is a powerful corrosive poison which when ingested causes inflammation or destruction of the gastro-intesternal mucous membrane. (Whitla, *Pharmacy, Materia Media and Therapeutics* Balliere, Tindall and Cox, London 1915)

[4] Cotyledon umbilicus; not described by Whitla.

[5] Phosphorus in large doses causes vomiting, purging and other signs of irritant presuring which may not show themselves until many hours after ingestion, later to subside and after a period of apparent recovery to return causing liver atrophy and failure.

[6] 4 Galium Mollage – a root of the Quinine family or Rubiacial – (Whitla)

consumption and that there was no need to worry about the future. By 1869 the Commissioners commented that clean bath water could now be supplied for each patient. The good times did not continue. As the number of patients increased the problem got worse. Not just the inconvenience of unhygienic sharing of bath water but serious public health effects. Typhoid fever occurred amongst patients and staff in 1873 & 1874. It became evident that surface wells and water from the river Frome would never supply a quantity sufficient for the hospital.

Laboratory examination of the water was advised and an attempt was made to persuade the Bristol Water Works to extend their mains to supply the hospital. The Chairman continued to be concerned not only about the water, but also the drainage and the milk supply. In 1874 it was considered that three deaths from enteric fever were due to contaminated water and the Commissioners recommended that a small-detached hospital should be built for the isolation and treatment of fevers. Water continued to be short during the summer months when surface water liable to contamination had to be used. The Commissioners complained bitterly that laboratory tests had not been carried out and threatened dire consequences if they continued to be neglected. No punitive action was necessary, however, because from 1877 the hospital was supplied with water by the Bristol Water Works. The tanks were finally charged from that source on 30th January of that year. Ten thousand gallons of water were available per day. No cases of typhoid occurred subsequently.

Dr Oxley-Stephens' work was not altogether in vain. How many staff realise that there is a one million gallon spring fed reservoir below our front lawn which dates from his time? The reservoir is a bricked over quarry, the roof being a series of arches and the location being near the roundabout on the front drive. The water from this quarry is now being used to supply the hospital laundry and boiler house with 7.0 million gallons a year making a saving of £11,000 per annum. These savings are now possible due to a new electric pump installation completed during March of this year at a cost of £4,000.

Dr Stephens continued to try to improve the social organisation of the hospital. There were country outings, Summer picnics, evening gatherings and dances, sometimes attended by visitors from outside the hospital together with ladies and gentlemen members of the family or friends of the officers who provided cheerful evenings "with comic songs, readings, recitations and humorous scenes in character, songs and lyrical pieces varied by overtures

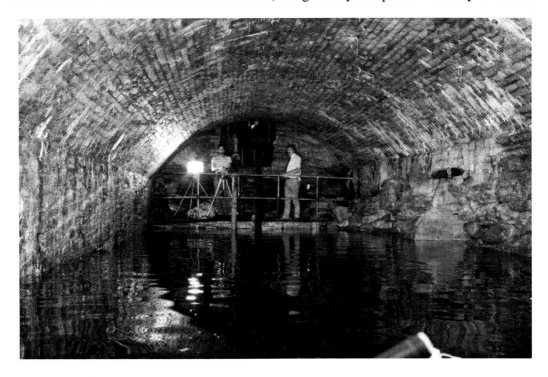

Figure 5 A recent exploration of the Reservoir

and other lively music performed on the pianoforte by the ladies and much enjoyed by the large numbers of patients." A pianoforte to be used in the Chapel or Hall had been presented by the Chairman of the Committee of Visitors.

By 1863 the asylum had been filled with patients much more quickly than was anticipated and already beds were being placed in a day room and in corridors on the female side of the hospital but overcrowding was a relief to the new Chairman, Frederick Terrell who was able to report a credit balance.

In 1865 the Commissioners urged enlargement of the hospital. In 1866 they opined that this could no longer be delayed. Dr Stephens pointed out that patients were accumulating at the rate of about 5% per annum and at the end of the first 5 years there was an accumulation of 49 patients. He thought that it seemed probable that this trend would continue and suggested that chronic and usually harmless patients could be transferred to the Union House. The Commissioners were of the view that no relief could be expected from that quarter. It was not until 1867 that the Committee obtained plans and estimates for an additional building to accommodate 15 males and 20 females. By the end of 1868 the additions to the buildings were nearly completed with the grant of some £3,000.00 to the Committee by the Council. When completed in 1869 the beds were in fact already filled and the medico-administrative problems continued.

In 1869 the Commissioners reported an extreme example of the sort of unsuitable cases of which Dr Stephens continued to complain. They agreed with him. "According to the Medical Journal the patients secluded for violence or dangerous propensities since last visit have been 9 men and 3 women, the latter on 5 occasions. One of the men referred to, deemed a dangerous lunatic was in August last sent to the asylum from Broadmoor" [opened in 1861] "as an insane convict whose sentence of penal servitude had expired. He is believed to have homicidal propensities, has threatened to injure the Superintendent and attendants and has been detected in concealing an offensive weapon. He has delusions as to poisonous drugs, uses foul language, is noisy day and night, and a source of alarm to the other inmates. He is reported to have been in several prisons and bears marks of the lash. For the above reasons we consider him a most unfit person to be retained as a patient in an ordinary asylum."

The first 10 years brought no stability to the hospital. The joy of liberation from St Peter's and the exuberance of escape from its ignoble conditions soon gave way to the realisation that the practical problems of increasing pressure for unsuitable admissions would not permit the establishment of a progressive liberal regime. Dr Stephens' zeal was gradually worn down by events. He could control neither the number, nor the quality of admissions, the infectious, the contagious, the demented, the behaviour–disturbed and imbeciles. The pathetically small cure rate soon made it obvious that the ideal hospital of 200 – 250 beds would not be achieved, the more especially when the Administration demanded that beds be kept full so that the cost of maintenance be reduced. They discovered that more and more patients could be looked after by less and less staff. The death rate was depressingly high. In spite of his assurances, the water supply remained a grave problem, in quality and quantity. The pressure grew increasingly during his superintendency and finally the matron, his long-term friend and colleague died. He could stand it no longer and in spite of 4 months sick leave, he retired in 1871.

The Committee appointed an assistant medical officer Dr W. Merrytt Hartlebury Day, in October 1870. He undertook "the arduous and responsible duties" of writing the annual medical report for that year, in which he recorded a yearly 10% increase in bed occupancy with continuing accumulation of a high percentage of epileptic and feeble persons.

In it he also wrote of the curious case of J.J.: "
    Among the deaths was that of one of the celebrities of the Asylum, known to the
    Visitors as the 'Man with the Wheel'. He had been an inmate from the first opening of

the establishment in 1861, having been transferred to the Asylum from St Peters Hospital. His delusional ideas related principally to his having a wheel perpetually working within his body, the revolution of the wheel giving him no rest night or day so that he had not slept for many years before his death. He said, "Tomorrow at ten o'clock the wheel will stop and I shall be in Heaven." As the Asylum clock was striking ten the following morning his Spirit took its flight.

Dr Stephens' illness was not fatal. He died in 1881 and is commemorated by a stained-glass window in the chancel of the hospital church. Dr Day died suddenly on a visit to Bath on 9th August 1871.

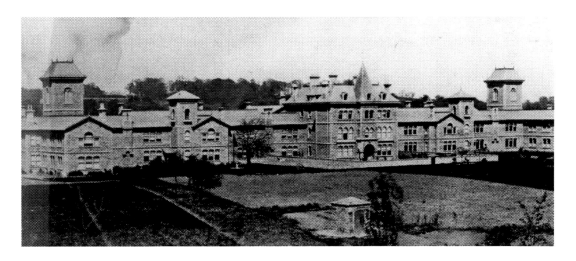

Figure 6 Another early photograph of the Asylum

From 1871 to The Lunacy Act of 1890

Mr George Thompson L.R.C.P. London, of the West Riding Wakefield Asylum took over from Dr Stephens on the 19th May 1871. The first of his reports was short, factual, non–contentious. From then onward they varied in quality and in quantity. For example, in January 1873 he described the Commissioners' 1872 report as highly favourable, although it was more critical than any other report to date. They complained of instances of restraint which had not been recorded, of a man wearing gloves to prevent self-injury whose name had not been entered, of the fact that there was no record in the case book of the deaths of two patients who died in the month prior to their visit, of several cases where the entries had not been made in the manner prescribed by the statute and of being unable to obtain any information about building on neighbouring land which they thought should have been prevented. These complaints were compounded by the failure to report the "most proper" dismissal of a nurse who was involved in a scuffle with a patient.

Such a spate of fault finding was not repeated and in general, throughout the decades leading up to the Lunacy Act 1890, the Commissioners tended to be moderate in their criticisms. Only once in 1882 did they adopt a tone which was threatening and menacing: "We have to report no alteration in the night supervision of epileptics and though there is on either side, a large dormitory which might be made available for almost continuous supervision, this has not been done. We repeat that should any patient die unattended from suffocation during an epileptic fit, the Medical Superintendent will be directly responsible for a death which might have been prevented."

The population of the City and County of Bristol in 1861, was 154,693. By 1871 it had risen to 183,298 and growing. Hospital overcrowding was increasing with the rise in the urban population, with a decrease of hospital death rate, with the more ready removal of cases to the asylum by relieving officers, and with the decreased resistance to admission from patients, from their relatives and their friends.

The number of patients exceeded accommodation by 1864 and enlargement of the asylum became inevitable. Six acres of land were purchased on the north of the estate and an extension was built to accommodate 13 men and 21 women. This was occupied in 1869 by which time it failed to deal with the then existing overcrowding; there were three in-patients more than the available space. Excess of admissions over discharges and deaths crept up relentlessly by ten per cent per annum so that by 1872, Dr Thompson's second year as Medical Superintendent, the Visitors described the hospital as inconveniently overcrowded and the Commissioners asserted that enlargement could no longer be delayed. In 1873 plans were prepared by Mr Hawton, the architect of the 1869 extension and although the hospital population kept on increasing, the provision of beds proceeded slowly through 1876 and 1877 to completion and occupation in 1878. This provided 60 male and 60 female beds. These extensions and increase in patient numbers made the existing dining hall and chapel too small for the hospital.

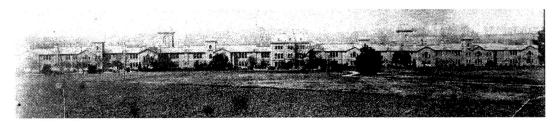

Figure 7 The Asylum after the 1870's extensions

A new church, built from 1879 to 1881, was opened for worship in August 1880. Plans for the conversion of the old chapel and the adjacent dining room into one room were sanctioned but the resulting Amusement Hall and the new dining hall were not completed until 1892. In 1880 there were again beds in the corridors and the Commissioners agreed that a further extension was needed but not until more land was acquired.

Mr Terrell retired in 1882 having been Chairman of the Visitors for 20 years. Charles Wathen was appointed in his stead. He inherited the most severe overcrowding to date, with beds on the floor and in corridors on the female wards. In his second year the hospital population rose to 460; he was obliged to arrange that 40 ladies be boarded out to Gloucester Asylum at 13 shillings [65p] per week and admission was restricted. In December 1884 Dr Thompson "found it necessary and expedient" to make a regulation under Sec 53 of the Lunatic Act 1853, which empowered the Medical Superintendent to refuse to admit any person suffering from specified contagious disease or anyone coming from a district in which such disease was present. This prevented the admission of patients suffering from fevers such as typhoid or from tuberculosis, curbed the Relieving Officers and reduced the number of chronic patients admitted.

Mr Wathen bought 6 acres of ground to the west of the estate bringing the total acreage to 40. In 1883, the Committee requested the Council for permission to enlarge the establishment to 750 beds and submitted plans with an estimate of £65,670–0–0d for the work. The Council referred the project back. It was 3 years before it was approved and returned to the Committee of Visitors.

Dr Thompson was an eccentric. He expressed more authoritative clinical opinions in his annual reports than was usual for a medical superintendent. He showed considerable interest in General Paralysis of the Insane (GPI). In 1871, he reported that 10 male patients and 1 female were admitted in an advanced stage of this condition. The following year he reported on 3 patients "who at the time of their admission presented unmistakable signs of the existence of the disease but who under the use of Calabar Bean (Physostigma Venenosum)[1] made rapid improvement. They were discharged and months later showed no tendency to relapse. So far as I am aware these are the first cases recorded of recovery from this fearful malady." Three years later he on two of these patients, 1 man and 1 woman; "The man's recovery was undoubtedly permanent" but with regard to the woman, "the incessant importunity and frequent rudeness of her friends caused her to be discharged before her convalescence was formally established and I fear she has relapsed."

The confidence with which the recovery was claimed in a then incurable disease is remarkable, but it could not be sustained. G.P.I. was amongst the commonest causes of death in asylums. Any claim of a curative agent would have been of world wide significance. He later expressed scepticism about the treatment and in 1888, when 21 of the 25 patients admitted with G.P.I. died. He then used Jaborandi[2] instead of Calabar "with about the same result." He continued to use Calabar Bean maintaining that it was probably beneficial in the early stages of General Paralysis, adding the recurrent complaint that cases are not presented for treatment at a sufficiently early stage to expect benefit to follow any mode of treatment "and until medical men outside asylums are trained to recognise this

---

[1] Calabar Bean: Dry seed yields Physostigmine or Eserine Sulphate, an alkaloid with profound paralytic effects. Sir William Whilta in "*Elements of Pharmacy, Materia Medica & Therapeutics* (1915)" relates that "it was long used by the West Africans as an ordeal for determining the guilt or innocence of suspected witches." Overdose causes death from respiratory failure.

[2] Jaborandi leaves are a source of Pilocarpine Nitrate which causes profuse salivation and sweating. Whilta (1915) ascribes to it a catholic array of uses: Brights Disease, pleural and peritoneal accumulations, asthma, pertussis, bronchitis, tonsillitis, laryngitis, diphtheria amenorrhoea, uterine affections, syphilis, atropine poisoning, chronic poisoning by iodine, lead & mercury, skin diseases such as prurigo and urticarea, baldness, toothache, enlarged glands, drunkenness.

disease in its earliest stage our tables of causes of death will present a large proportion of deaths in asylums as being due to this sad disease."

The other main asylum illnesses were epilepsy, phthisis and other infectious diseases. Cases of enteric and typhoid fever recurred until the water supply was connected to the City mains in 1876.

The nursing staff received little mention in the medical reports. In 1882 the Head Attendant was dismissed, no cause was recorded. Miss Yeames a senior nursing officer died of fulminating tuberculosis complicating Typhoid Fever in 1875. A female nurse was dismissed in 1871 for pushing a patient; three nurses in '73 for breaking the rules. In the same year was recorded the case of an old attendant and faithful servant (William F) who was bitten on the thumb by a patient Samuel C "labouring under erysipelas." The thumb sloughed and had to be removed. The attendant recovered and was granted a liberal annuity by the Council.

The medical superintendent's 1875 report contained a description, not without humour, of the case of E.W. In 1863 he refers to this patient, a woman who gave rise to much anxiety, because of an attempt which she made to commit suicide by swallowing the contents of a domino box and a number of pebbles which when recovered weighed fourteen ounces. In 1875 he wrote:

> This year she has performed a feat which puts her former one entirely in the shade. She was admitted for the third time in June last. On the 21st of July she got possession of a number of iron screws used in the ward for securing the window shutters, of these she swallowed thirteen before breakfast. A cursory examination showed that her own statement was true; the contents of her stomach could be made to rattle so as to be heard across a large room. The screws were 2⅝ inches in length ½ inch thick having a square head for the application of a key and a collar projecting ⅛ inch from the main body of the screw. Thirteen similar screws weighed 24½ ounces Troy weight. One screw that had not been swallowed weighed 730 grains. She retained this mass of solid iron with very little inconvenience except spasmodic pains. On the 6th September one screw weighing 700 grains passed from the bowels. Since then she has passed 4 more screws. I give the dates and the weights:- October 19th, 665 grains; November 26th, 645 grains; November 27th, 645 grains; and December 3rd, 555 grains. This case is certainly an extraordinary one and calls for no further comment.

The Annual Report for 1876 describes "The last of the case of E.W.: The remainder (of the screws) were got rid of by the 4th of February in the year just closed and a month afterwards she was transferred to the Asylum of her own county. The 13 shutter screws weighed 24½ ounces"

Dr Thompson's rather pompous mode of presentation, as well as the content of his reports, gave some indication of his selfesteem. He anticipated that his opinions would be widely read. "It will therefore not be out of place, perhaps, to say something of some of the means used for treating the patients medicinally. I should say at once, then, that chloral,[1] bromide of potassium[2] and cannabis Indica[3] – those dreadful destroyers of brain function – are not used in this Asylum. But during the year a new weapon has been added to our armoury which promises to be of great service in the treatment of acute, chronic and recurrent mania. I refer to the hypobromate of hyoscine[4]. Given in doses of from 1/200th to 1/60th of a grain by mouth or injected beneath the skin, the effect, especially on the latter class of cases is simply marvellous. Where the tendency of such persons (a very common one) is to destroy their clothing and property generally, the new drug most peremptorily puts a stop to it. But the hyoscine should on no account be given to an epileptic, as that condition known as status

---

[1] Chloral Hydrate: Hypnotic & Sedative
[2] Bromide of potassium: a sedative used as such and in epilepsy up to the 1940's. Chronic use led to symptoms of bromisim with confusion and worsening of mental symptoms.
[3] Cannabis Indica: "a true narcotic" (Whitla). Intoxication causes excitement followed by sleep and coma.
[4] Hypodromide of Hyoscine or Scopolomine: a powerful sedative and hypnotic. (Whitla)

epilepticus[5] is at once induced in a dangerous degree. I find that small doses of aconite[6] and antimony[7] together or alone are of great service in the treatment of the ordinary morose epileptic. The fits are reduced in number and the temper and manners and intelligence are improved all round." In 1882, he described epilepsy as the most dangerous and most hopeless of cases, representing 90 cases out of 420 in-patients in 1885 of whom 12 - 15% were actively suicidal.

On hospital privileges and considered extravagances he wrote: "When the report of 1876 was printed, one of your number drew my attention to the apparent extravagance in spending £95 in this article of luxury (tobacco). I then compared the cost here with that incurred in other Asylums and I found that the amount spent in all Asylums per head counting men and women varied from 6s.9d. [34p] in one to 10½d [4p] in another. The cost here was 3s.1d [15½p]. Almost seventy men consumed this tobacco and many of them were general paralytics, epileptics and so forth. Besides many were "loafers" who while unwilling to work in the garden "curried favour" by sweeping up the crumbs after each meal, and so assured an allowance of tobacco. These I struck off the list, and by keeping a strict watch on it, have reduced the amount by two-thirds so that while the cost is reduced to a third, no one so far as I can see, is any the worse for it and in many instances the withdrawal of such a vicious habit has been followed by a marked brightening of the mind of the patient. There are many patients, suffering from nervous 'breakdown' who probably have been helped to that dire condition by too free indulgence in a most baneful habit. The 'hardship' of leaving off is a sentimental matter entirely..." This lengthy opinion is followed next year by: "I refer to this question once more because the critics have had a turn at me. If I say that the expenditure on this item (tobacco) was £95 in 1886, £31 in 1888 and £27 in 1889 and that everybody is all the better for the change, I may satisfy the critics. Soon I hope not to mention it, because I hope it will disappear as an item on the accounts of this asylum."

In 1883 Dr Thompson had a similar moral victory when beer ceased to be an article of ordinary diet. He had long maintained that beer was of no dietetic value "or if it had any, that value was counterbalanced by the deleterious effect, moral and physical which it had. The patients drank the ordinary amount allowed as a matter of course, and were not benefited by it. Those who were expected to do work got an extra allowance and were all the more discontented with their lot. No extra work could be got out of anybody unless extra beer was allowed. The nurses and female servants seldom drank it, but received no compensation for the abstinence; while the male attendants were often "the worse" for what they consumed."

Beer was no longer sent to the wards and a payment in lieu was made to staff. Each paid man received £4 and each paid woman £2 per annum instead of a beer allowance "and insobriety is now very conspicuous by its absence."

His pomposity can be judged from almost two pages of report and comment on water heating and fire control in his annual report of 1884: "As to women firemen I have strong opinions on that point. The nurse mentioned in my report... said in reply to a question (as to what she would do in case of fire) that she would send for assistance – meaning male assistance, of course. I have Mr Superintendent Wingfield's authority to say that in his opinion, it is the wisest determination she or any other woman could arrive at; and that if I found that any woman thought that she could put out a fire or even arrest one, I had better recommend her to get employment elsewhere."

His imperious tone was not confined to his dealings with nursing underlings as can be seen by his attitude to the highest authority in the land described by John Bird in his unpublished paper "Madness, Crime and Politics" which I quote with his permission. "For threatening to shoot the Prince of Wales, William John Donne was committed to Bristol Lunatic Asylum on 2nd February 1884. He was confirmed as a criminal lunatic under warrant to the Home

---

[5] Status epilepticus: a succession of epileptic fits recurring one after another, without regaining of consciousness.
[6] Aconite: a cardiac sedative, diaphoretic and diuretic. (Whitla)
[7] Antimony: an element resembling Arsenic in many ways was used "to reduce the force of the pulse" as a diaphoretic and as an emetic.(Whitla)

Secretary, Sir William Harcourt, on the basis of the 1840 Insane Prisoners Act (3&4 Vict c54). He remained incarcerated in asylums until his death despite many attempts to prove his sanity, in Bristol until 1888, in Abergavenny until 1897 and finally in Broadmoor until he died on the 2nd of April 1902 aged 51. In common with many criminal lunatics he never stood trial. His case raises important issues concerning the relationships between crime and insanity, between politics and insanity and gives some insights into the working of the asylum, the Home Office and the legal system."

Donne believed that the Prince had mesmerised him by virtue of his power as head of the Freemasons and compelled him to act in certain ways. When his delusions were not touched on he conversed sensibly, although he was restless and excitable at times, and again was irritable and threatening.

His case aroused considerable local interest and there were several attempts to achieve his discharge. In May 1885, Donne wrote to the Home Office requesting his release. The Medical Superintendent opined that he was as insane as when he was admitted. In September 1886, Donne's solicitor wrote to the Home Office on the behest of the Mayor of Bristol and of some of the Visitors of the Asylum enquiring about the possibility of release. They were concerned about the legality of his detention but did not feel justified in discharging him having regard to the fact that he was detained under Order of the Home Office. The Home Office asked for a report from Dr.Thompson and he replied.

The request contained in your letter that I will report to you on the mental condition of W.J.Donne a lunatic prisoner on remand, now an inmate of this asylum, places me, I respectfully submit, in a rather awkward position. By the order of your predecessor in office, Sir W.V.Harcourt, I am constituted Mr Donne's jailer; now you wish to make me his judge. That is a position to which I do not aspire, nor do I think it is fair for me to assume.

The lunatic in question, besides being an insane prisoner on remand, has had an inquisition held upon him by a Master of Lunacy who found him insane and he is therefore a lunatic was in Chancery. As such he is visited twice a year by one of the Lord Chancellor's Visitors in Lunacy, the last visit was recently made by Sir Charles Crichton-Browne, MD who apparently has made no official report to the Court or I should most probably have heard of it.

As I strongly object to allow myself to be constituted an ultimate court of appeal I would, with due respect, suggest that the report now asked for should be procured from some medical man, a known expert on the knowledge of lunacy, but unconnected with this asylum, say Dr Wade of the Somerset County Asylum at Wells, or Mr F Hurst Craddock of the Gloucester County Asylum at Cirencester. A report coming from such an independent source would surely be free from any suspicion of bias and more satisfactory on the whole.

I have the honour to be Sir
Your very obedient servant......."

To this the Home Office reply was "I am directed by the Secretary of State to say that he regrets to have received your letter of the 9th inst with regard to the care of the Criminal Lunatic William Donne. It stresses that the Superintendent is shirking his responsibilities, but that the Home Office will follow his recommendation to consult the Lord Chancellor's Visitors. Dr Thompson by his position as a medical man who is not at the same time running a prison and added, "I am pleased to find that you have adopted the suggestion I made in my letter of the 9th inst that an independent opinion... be obtained from the Lord Chancellor's Visitors Office."

"I would say that I do not see in what way it is proved that I have shrunk from my duty as Medical Officer and Superintendent of the Asylum. In the case under consideration my opinion is formed and it takes a very decided form too... it is not out of disrespect of the Home Office that I decline to express that opinion but rather... because I have no desire to be at one and the same time Mr Donne's jailer and judge."

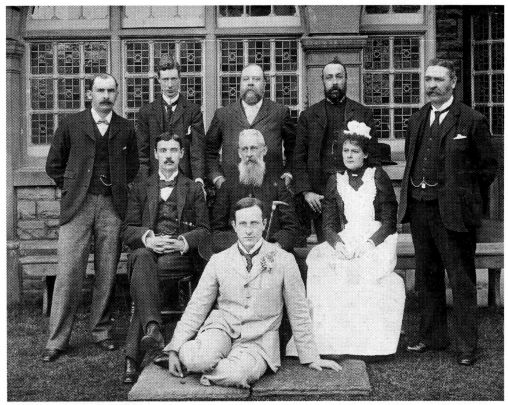

Arthur Orme	Henry Robert Withycombe	George Thompson M.D.	Henry A Benham M.D.	D Travers Burgess
Clerk & Steward	Clerk of Works	Medical Superintendent	First Assistant M.O.	Clerk to the Visitors

Alderman Charles Wathen   Rev. James Fountaine[*]   Julia A Crook
Mayor & Chairman of Visiting Committee   Chaplain   House Keeper

Frederick L.H. Brown   2nd Assistant M.O.

Figure 8 Senior Staff in the 1880's

There was no answer to this except an internal Home Office rhetorical sigh of exasperation: "Is this to be put up with?"

The Chairman commented on Dr. Thompson's poor state of health in 1884. His erratic behaviour continued. Almost in desperation Mr Wathen appointed Dr Harry Benham as an Assistant Medical Officer and sent Dr.Thompson on 6 months leave during which time he went on a long sea-voyage with no permanent benefit to his health.

When building work started in November 1886, Thompson was unable to cope with the ensuing activity. There were 270 workmen employed on structural alterations and additions which included the building of two large wings each to accommodate 117 patients projecting forward from the original building with 2 smaller wings each of 40 places. Also approved were the workshops and a mortuary. By the end of 1888 the 2 large wings (2 x 117patients) and 2 small wings (2 x 42 patients) were finished whilst the old dormitories which were undergoing reconstruction to serve as their day rooms were not ready until the following year, 1889. Temporary offices, stores, kitchens etc were provided in 1889 to replace the administration block, which was demolished in 1890. The chaos surrounding the demolition and reconstruction of the central block was unimaginable. Alderman Wathen steered the hospital through this major reconstruction, which continued over 8 years. This entailed a massive upheaval including Dr Thompson having to vacate his hospital house and find outside accommodation whilst bemoaning "the extensive pulling down and building up." In

---

[*] In this photograph, the central figure has always been identified as Thompson, with Bentham behind and Fountaine to the right. Now a relative of Fountaine has made it irrefutable that the central figure is Fountaine, so if Thompson is shown he must be behind Fountaine (previously identified as Benham) and Benham is as shown (previously identified as Fountaine).

his last, sad annual report he wrote of the admission of a more and more hopeless class of patient which included 16 general paralytics, 15 epileptics over 60 years of age and 7 congenital idiots. Of the hospital population of 508 patients he considered that "out of this vast concourse of effete human material, there are altogether 15 cases which present a reasonable prospect of recovery."

In 1890 the year of the Lunacy Act, major building operations continued on the site. The 270 workmen engaged on the erection of the new administration block went on strike, postponing the completion of the building for many months. At the same time there was an epidemic of influenza which attacked the nursing staff, many of whom were prostrated by the disease. Dr Thompson was depressed and broken in health. After nearly 20 years as medical superintendent he retired on medical grounds in June 1890. He died later in Stanley Royd Hospital.

Alderman Wathen was knighted and continued as Chairman.

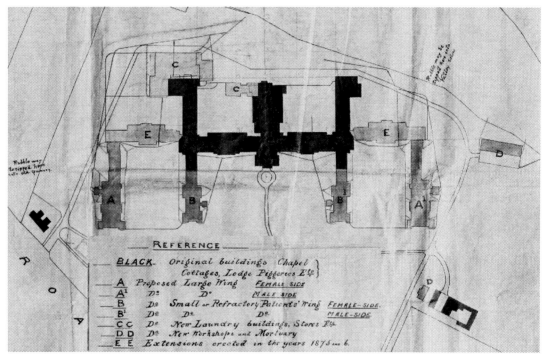

Figure 9 The Alterations 1870 - 1890

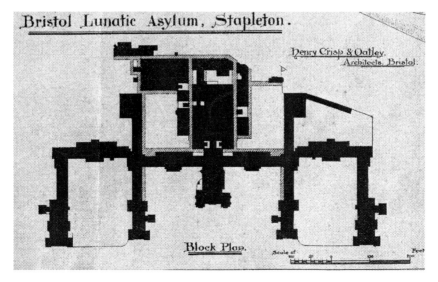

Figure 10 A plan from 1890's

23

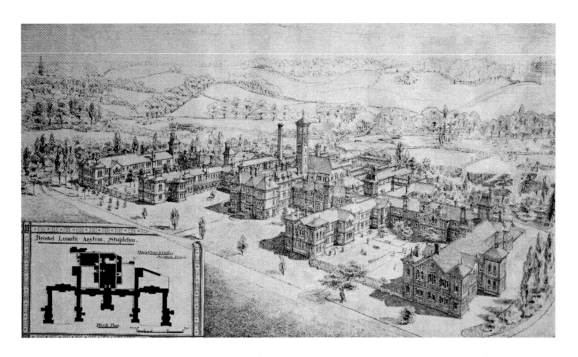

Figure 11   Bristol Asylum 1890's

From 1890 to the Outbreak of World War One

The final decade of the 19th Century began under new medical direction.

After 19 years as medical superintendent, to the plaudits of the Commissioners, Dr Thompson was liberally pensioned and the second Benham brother, Dr Harry (1890–1904) assumed his mantle. His older brother William had served Bristol Lunatic Asylum as assistant medical officer for 2½ years from 1872, after which "his hopes of promotion were more than realised when he received the highly lucrative post of Physician in Chief of the Chilean State Asylum." Harry, too, was a high flyer. He inherited a hospital in chaos.

The building works were at a standstill caused by a strike of the workmen engaged in the construction of the new administrative and ward blocks. When they returned to work late in spring (1890), their action was emulated by a dissatisfied male nursing staff. They all withdrew their labour, except Male Nurse White who was off sick and the Head Attendant, and were promptly sacked.

These problems were not mentioned by the Chairman in his annual report but Dr Benham referred to the staff action as "an experience... unique amongst similar institutions in this country." He was happy and relieved that no casualty had occurred "although it occasioned great anxiety to all connected with the administration of the asylum." The Chaplain was more positive, simply recording that the exodus of male attendants "caused the Choir to be at present in a less efficient state than formerly."

The vacant nursing places were immediately filled and replaced by new staff who, said the Chairman, "performed their duties efficiently and in a satisfactory manner." This stimulated the padre to report a marked improvement in the chanting since the Cathedral Psalter introduced "a much needed change", and enabled those who could read to take an active part in the service.

Apart from this aside, there was no comment on the effect, which the turmoil must have had on patients. It was nearly one hundred years before nurses again took serious industrial action

Dr Benham inherited many other problems. The new Lunacy Act came into force in May (1890) and caused considerable additional work. The women's side of the hospital was nearly full. Then an epidemic of influenza caused concern in the Spring.

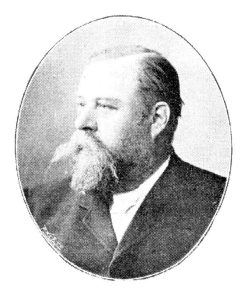

Figure 12 Dr Henry A. Benham - Medical Superintendent 1890 - 1904

The population of Bristol continued to grow, rising to 226,510 in 1888 and as it grew so did the numbers of admissions. Dr Benham complained of the incurability of the patients unloaded on to the Asylum by the Poor Law . He claimed that he had 120 epileptics under his care and like Dr Thompson he too considered it unfortunate that his Asylum should have more of "this dangerous and almost incurable class than any other asylum." Most epileptics – almost one-third of the Asylum population had no reasonable prospect of recovery. In fact in 1892, he complained that only 7 male and 10 female patients under his care had any chance of improvement.

In his early days, the Commissioners were critical of Dr Benham. In 1891 they asked that each patient should have a separate drinking vessel at meal times so that 5 or 6 of them need not drink from one mug. They complained that the workshops were too small. Suicide caution cards were introduced in accordance with the their advice. Benham thought them of little use, since they did not require that patients be in the constant sight of attendants throughout the day and anyhow 19 out of 22 male attendants had less than 3 months service. They recommended that tell tale clocks should be installed to test attendant's vigilance and so he installed them
Within a couple of years they changed their tune and spoke of his energetic management. Dr Benham himself was enthusiastic about the eventful year of 1892 and enumerated all the exciting additions to the hospital. The Administration block was completed as were the new dining room, the amusement hall, the kitchen, the stewards stores and offices, the housekeepers room, the servants quarters, the bakery, the surgery, the porters lodge, the visiting and admission room for patients and the new laundry which now meant that he could provide each patient with 2 clean shirts per week.

Work on the Administration and Residential block was scheduled to take 2 years to finish when started in 1891. In this year patient numbers reached 550; the new dining and amusement halls were in use.

In January 1893, Alderman Sir Charles Wathen, the Chairman reported that all alterations and extensions were complete including the entire reconstruction of the administration department. He expressed satisfaction and relief that no patient had been injured in consequence of the building operations. He purchased 8 acres of land on the side of the road opposite from the hospital.
He died in 1893 after 12 tumultuous years in the Chair.

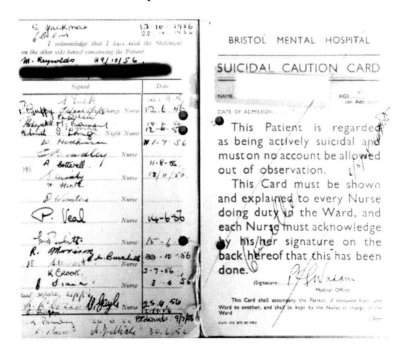

Figure 13 Suicide Caution Card - introduced in 1890's, still in use 1950's

Alderman Charles Hoskins Low took his place. Nine further acres of land were bought in 1892 and in 1894 the property known as Stapleton Mill was purchased by the committee. "The purchase" said the Chairman "rounds off the asylum estate and will enable the part of the estate adjoining the mill to be better utilised."

Building works continued and were administratively and clinically intrusive but they proceeded less frenetically. All the land at the back of the workhouse was acquired in 1900. The Bungalow (isolation hospital) was built and eight further acres were purchased in 1902.

Educational improvements were taking place. Lectures by medical officers were being given to attendants on first aid and on nursing. By 1895, the Handbook for Attendants of the Insane was published and the certificate of the Medico-Psychological Association (MPA) first awarded in 1886, had been gained by 18 staff members who thereby became entitled to the MPA badge and a gratuity of £2 on completion of each subsequent year of service.

In addition to 30 staff members passed the First Aid examination of the St. John's Ambulance Association. By 1896 all Charge Nurses and Attendants held Certificate of the Medico-Psychological Association. Uniform was introduced for female nursing staff. An infirmary ward was organised.

Tell-tale clocks were supplied on the wards, an electric fire alarm was installed. Locked boxes for cutlery were ordered and a new type of towel roller was introduced in the bathrooms.

More patients were at work and one of the Assistant Medical Officers organised a string band, the first since the strike.

A laboratory was equipped together with photographic facilities. These were used to photograph the patients as well as other things.

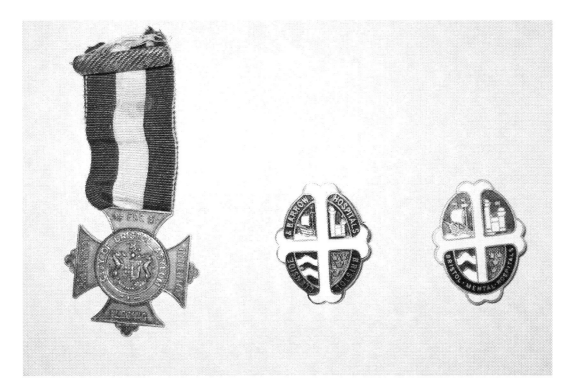

Figure 14   Nurse Badges of Medico-Psychological Association & Glenside Hospital

The quality of admissions in 1893 was as poor as ever. Bed numbers rose to 653. Nothing could be done to restrict or to control admissions. Dr Benham explained that although some of the admissions might be equally well treated in an imbecile ward in the workhouse the Union authorities had no inducement to make provision for them owing to their receiving a capitation fee of 4/- (20p) for every case under asylum treatment, they can keep any patient chargeable to them in an asylum at no additional cost to themselves. Dr Benham considered that this should apply equally to cases kept in the Union House under Sec 25of the Lunacy Act. But it didn't. He tested his thesis by transferring to the workhouse 9 men and 9 women under this Section. He thought that it would be more profitable to the Union to retain them there than to admit them to the Asylum. But nobody listened. The dying, the demented and the dangerous came in relentless numbers. Overcrowding was either present or threatening. The male wards if not bulging with Bristol patients, had lodgers, patients from other hospitals. Complaints from patients from Denbigh Asylum were so distressing to the Commissioners that at their suggestion they were provided with newspapers, periodicals and picture bibles in Welsh until such time as they returned home in 1895. They were then replaced by 60 Londoners who complained about the niggardly tobacco allowance. Justifiably, said the Commissioners, and it was increased.

In February 1895, Dr Benham reported that the extensions were finally finished and opened, comprising of the Committee room, the new Superintendents house, the assistant medical officers apartments, the patients' visiting and receiving rooms, the mess rooms for nurses, attendants and servants, a room for photography and a room for pathological research. Wards 2 and 10 were converted into hospital wards each with a padded room and having additional nursing staff at night.

Already the female beds were again full. A further 30 acres of land were bought and by 1897 plans for the accommodation of up to 1,000 patients were being considered. The Commissioners were urging that female beds be built. The extension of the City boundaries imposed by the Bristol Corporation Act 1897 added 80,000 more inhabitants to the City and laid on the Committee the necessity of providing for 139 additional patients, 65 males and 74 females. It was hoped that the amalgamation of Parishes into one central Authority might ease the pressures on the hospital but that was not to be. It added to them. The extra 150 beds from newly planned wards 17,18,19 and 20 would not be ready until 1900.

The unsatisfactory admission pattern continued to be complicated by the reception of groups of patients from other hospitals. Fifty-four (54) men and 65 women were received from the Gloucester County Asylum, (Wotton) in 1897, plus 11 men and 9 women from Somerset County Asylum (Wells) to which hospital two groups of 30 men were returned later in the year. They were replaced by 30 men from London under contract with the Asylums Committee of the London County Council (L.C.C). None of these were hopeful cases and the helpless and incurable continued to pour in.

In spite of these problems the Commissioners still referred to the very favourable conditions in the hospital with quiet and general contentment prevailing.

Dr Benham complained that he couldn't win. Depending on current public sentiment he was blamed for keeping people too long in hospital or for discharging them too early.

Admissions in 1898, rose to 216, with a 55% increase in those over the age of 65. The ratio of staff to patients, 1 to 11 was considered adequate until in 1899, when on the outbreak of the Boer War, 16 male attendants were called to the colours so that replacement staff which followed the strike of 10 years previously, again suffered a depletion of nearly one-half of its number.

By the end of 1900, the buildings sanctioned in May 1897 were completed. In 1901 the Night Nurses annexe and the isolation hospital were occupied and Wards 17, 18, 19, and 20 were completed. The new dining hall for males had a theatrical stage built in it.

The hospital population reached 920. Dr Benham was feeling the strain. In December 1901 he was granted 6 months leave. He returned in July feeling much better and had to deal with an epidemic of septic pneumonia which caused 10 deaths in the female epileptic ward, 7 of them after only 3 days illness. The cause was unknown; "it disappeared as suddenly as it came." It was preceded in the spring by an outbreak of scarlet fever which affected 4 men and 7 women, including 1 nurse, all of whom were treated in the new isolation hospital and recovered.

Dr Benham's health was failing. He attended to his duties up to 14th September 1904 when he was found dead in his office chair.

His death was unexpected and a gloom fell over the whole establishment. His name is perpetuated in the Benham armchair, a sturdy piece of furniture which he is said to have designed when few chairs were available. They continued in use until the 1950's.

He introduced billiards in 1884, a new croquet pitch in 1892 and a bowling green in 1896.

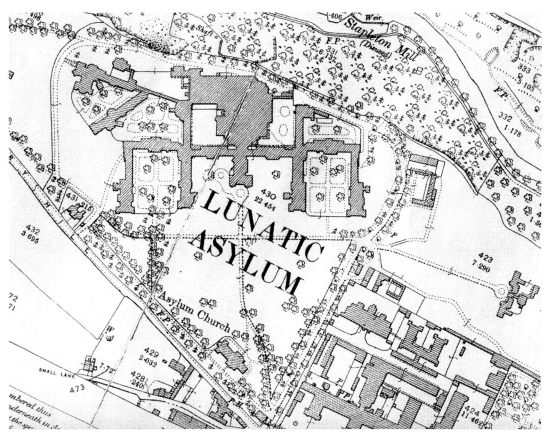

From 1904 Ordnance Survey map.

Figure 15 Bristol Lunatic Asylum 1904

(This shows the asylum before the additional male wards were built on right end)

The Beaufort War Hospital 1915 – 1919:

"No more glorious memorial."

Dr Benham was succeeded by Dr J Vincent Blatchford his first Assistant Medical Officer who inherited the medical supervision of a hospital of 951 patients (419 male, 532 female) an increase of 116 over the previous year.

In 1904, there were 355 admissions (143 male, 213 women). Overcrowding worsened on the male side and a scheme for extension of accommodation was designed to bring the number of male beds up to 450. This plan was altered in 1906 to provide for 90 new beds instead of the previously proposed 45. Building began in 1907 and was completed in 1909. The operations "added greatly to the duties and responsibilities of the medical superintendent, officers and attendants."

At this time annual reports became dull and routinely factual giving little information and conveying little of the contemporary atmosphere. In 1910 the Commissioners asked that more particulars be recorded in the case books relating to the medical and surgical treatment, especially in the case of injury. In 1911 they criticised the way the medical registers were kept and recommended that more attention be paid to the examination of the mental health of patients.

The discontinuance of a stock bottle of aperient on each ward was recommended. It may have disappeared. This is not recorded. If it did it made a comeback and persisted into the forties.

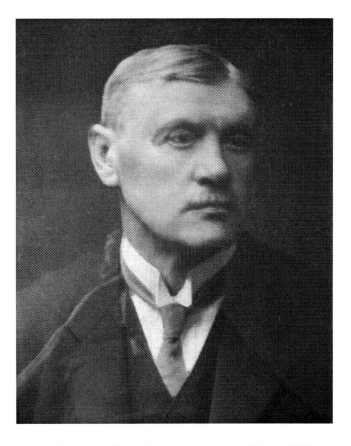

Figure 16 R J. V. Blatchford Medical Superintendent 1904 - 1924

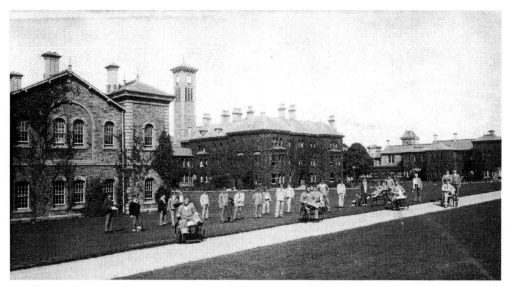

Figure 17 Patients in front of the Beaufort War Hospital

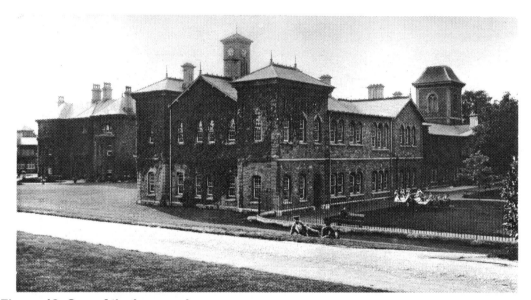

Figure 18 One of the 'squares'.

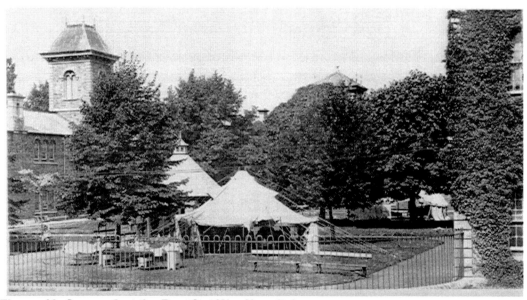

Figure 19 Square 2 at the Beaufort War Hospital

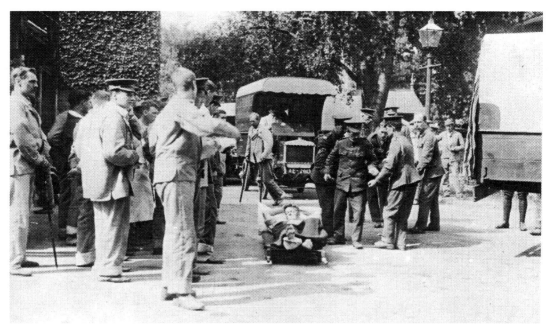

Figure 20 Arrival of patients

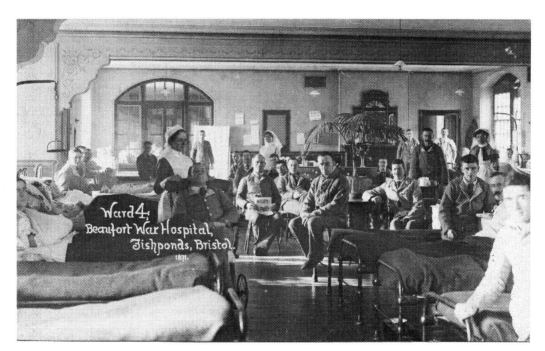

Figure 21 Ward 4

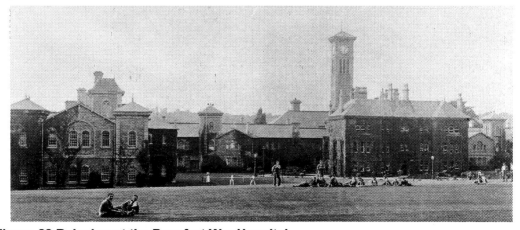

Figure 22 Relaxing at the Beaufort War Hospital

Dr Blatchford was interested in the farm, was proud that nearly all the garden produce required was grown on the estate and that the surplus of pork showed a good profit. Again and again he reported on satisfactory garden results and their contribution to the hospital economy. The Commissioners agreed and commended the attention given to patient diet. They said that this and "the way that patients were allowed to express their grievances to the Committee is one of the great features in the administration of this asylum and contributes considerably to the contentment which prevails."

Dr Blatchford prepared his annual report by precisely repeating the same pattern year by year. Not much new was happening so it was difficult to find anything new to say. He juggled words around so that his "special thanks (to staff) for loyal and willing services" in 1910 became " thanks for loyal and valuable services cheerfully given" in 1911. This probably reflected the fact that the pay of married male staff had gone up and "they were more contented"!

There were too few female nurses and night cover was inadequate. The size of the wards (eg. 95 beds in ward 12) was causing severe strain in caring for so many "troublesome type patients in one mass." Arrangements for alteration of these large wards were under consideration but came to nothing. World War I intervened.

Up to and during 1914 all appeared to be remarkably normal. On May 5th of that year the Commissioners expressed concern that the thick soup served for dinner was not popular, "a good deal of it being left" and thought that it "would probably be more appetising if it were made up as a stew."

The Chaplain writing his annual report on December 31st 1914 made no mention of the war that had started. On February 6th 1915 the Medical Superintendent reported that "in August last nearly 50 per cent of the male staff were called up for active service, their places were filled temporarily by persons with no previous experience... without inconvenience to the patients." The office of Junior Medical Officer was difficult to fill because of the war and other circumstances. He noted that the cost of provisions, clothing etc. had greatly increased the expenditure but that he hoped "to tide over the present crisis without having to make any extra charge for the maintenance of patients." The charges "necessarily caused some little anxiety at times."

Alderman George Pearson presented his Chairman's Annual Report on 27th March 1915.
> Your Committee have to report that in consequence of the war three married attendants and twenty-one single attendants have been ordered to rejoin their regiments. The vacancies thus caused have been filled by temporary men, who have been subject to a week's notice and have not been placed on the permanent staff. ....
> Your Committee regret to report that three of the attendants, named Wallace Ede, Frederick Buttle and Stewart Alexander Laverty, have been killed whilst on active service, and they desire to record their appreciation of the services which these men so readily rendered to their country. ...
> Early in February last your Committee received an intimation from the Board of Control that the War Office would in all probability require some additional beds for wounded soldiers when the new Armies went to the Front, and they hoped by clearing some Asylums entirely of their present patients and distributing them in other Institutions that 15,000 beds could be supplied by this means. ...
> The Board of Control further stated that after very careful consideration they came to the conclusion that a most determined effort should be made to supply the War Office, if the necessity arises, with the number of beds asked for, realising at the same time that such a scheme would necessarily involve over-crowding of patients, upsetting of arrangements, risks of accidents and other untoward events, and inconvenience and additional anxiety upon the staffs, but they felt in such a grave national crisis these difficulties must be faced, and no doubt will be cheerfully borne. ...Your Committee readily decided to give the proposals their hearty support. The Bristol City Asylum – one of the suggested vacating Asylums – was accordingly offered and accepted by

the War Office, and it was decided that the following Asylums should be grouped with Bristol, viz :- Dorset Asylum, Wilts Asylum, Somerset Wells Asylum, Somerset Cotford Asylum, Devon Asylum. Exeter Asylum, Plymouth Asylum. Cornwall Asylum. ... Your Committee therefore conferred with the above-named receiving Asylums, and arrangements were duly made for the removal of the patients to those Institutions. Considerable alterations were necessary to equip the Asylum as a Military Hospital, and acting upon the authority of the Board, which they received from the War Office, your Committee invited tenders for carrying out the work, which is accordingly being done at the War Office expense.

Your Committee have very carefully considered the details of reimbursement which the War Office undertake to make to receiving and vacating Asylums, and your Committee will continue to do all in their power to assist the Board of Control and the War Office in the work which they have been called upon to perform. ... The Committee will take the opportunity from time to time of visiting the patients at the Asylum to which they have been transferred. ...

The Bristol Asylum will be known as The Beaufort War Hospital during the time it is in use as a Military Hospital.

Alderman Pearson's next annual report was on 2nd April 1921.

Our first attempt to glean information about the role of the Bristol Mental Hospital Fishponds in the First World War drew a blank from the Curator of the RAMC Historical Museum Aldershot, who having visited the Muniment Room at the RAMC College, Millbank, advised that: "In the World War I Medical Services General History is a list of hospitals used including lunatic asylums and other buildings. However, in the Bristol area only the Poor Law Infirmary (King Edward VII Wing), Redmaids Secondary School, Poor Law Institution Southmead and a private house (Bishops Knoll) is shown as occupied by 2 (Southern) General Hospitals RAMC (TA) comprising 200 beds officers, 1742 beds soldiers."

Nor was much archival evidence left behind. We found a note book with "The Gallipoli Campaign" written on the cover and then, exasperatingly, all the leaves torn out. There is a letter dated December 2nd 1916 - 3 weeks after King George's visit – in which Robert Jones writing from the Automobile Club on behalf of General Birsell informs Colonel Blatchford of a gift of £1000 from the King Manuel of Portugal to be expended on orthopaedic appliances and on alterations to start curative workshops plus approval for £200 to be spent on electrical equipment and £250 for an X Ray outfit.

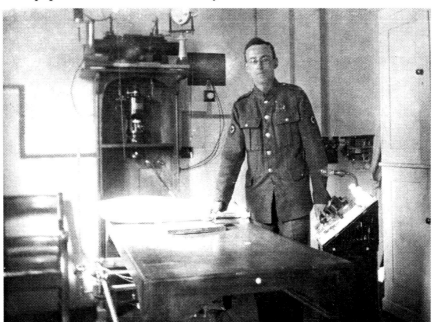

Figure 23 X-Ray department at Beaufort War Hospital

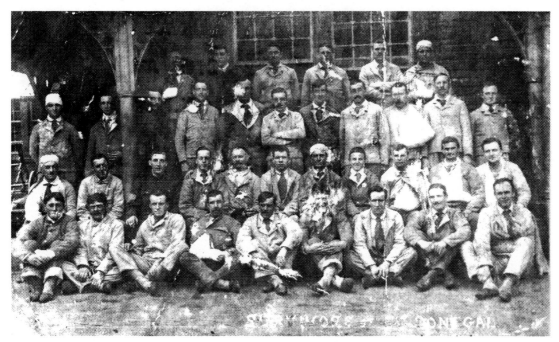

Figure 24 Survivors of the S.S.Donegal 23rd April 1917

The Museum has also received a donation from the son of Private J Clement of the 2nd Battalion of the Royal Scots Fusiliers of the above photograph of the survivors of the S.S.Donegal, a hospital ship torpedoed in April 1917 on its way from Boulogne to Southampton. His father is fourth from the right in the front row.

I am afraid I do not know too much about it but I will tell you what I do know.
My father, fourth from the right, in the front row. The one unfortunately which is somewhat scratched. He was 12787 Private J Clement of the 2nd Battalion Royal Scots Fusiliers. The SS Donegal was a hospital ship returning form France with wounded troops, I believe Boulogne to Southampton, when she was torpedoed by a German U-Boat. The survivors were picked up by another ship which was sailing for Avonmouth, which is why the men came to Glenside.

You may be interested a little in my father as I feel after what he did at that time, in this day and age, he would have had about 6 VC's, but not so then. Father was a Scotsman born in very poor circumstances in the Ayrshire hills which used to be a coal mining area. He left school at 10 years of age and worked on a farm. After war was declared in August 1914 he joined the Royal Scots Fuiliers at their barracks at Ayr (now demolished) on the second day of the war. Exactly when he went to France I am not sure, but it was early on and he was an old 'Contemptables' at 19, although he was always loath to admit it. He fought at many battles, including the disastrous battle of Loos, 1915. Out of one thousand men in his battalion he was one of only fifty survivors in one days fighting. He was at the Battle of Ypres, 1916, and he survived that. On the Menin Gate at Ypres there are approx two thousand names from his regiment alone. He also fought at Poperinge, the big battle at Bapaume, Bethune, St Quentin Armentiers, Hazelroack, Arras, Amien and Abbeville and he was also at Beauvais in early 1918 when our troops halted and turned the Germans back from Paris and possibly many more smaller actions. During this time he was wounded 5 times and gassed; suffered badly with trench foot and was badly scolded by boiling hot water not to mention the sinking of the SS Donegal. That was the third time he was wounded. His pay was seven shillings a week, of which he always sent three shillings and sixpence to his father. At the battle of Ypres the dead were piled fifteen high, which the attacking men had to climb over before they could get out of the trenches. The horror of that battle recoils on me and I was a tank driver for four years.

Fishponds was urgently called into use in 1915 when the other Bristol hospitals could not cope with the increasing influx of casualties from the Western Front. It was converted at War Office expense and provided 1460 beds. Very little notice of occupation was given to the asylum managers and even less warning of transfer to patients and their relatives. For example on 10th March 1915 the Secretary of the Board of Control wrote to JFB Esq.:

> Mrs P.L.B.
> I beg to inform you that an Order under Section 59 of the Lunacy Act, 1890, for the transfer of this patient to Wilts Asylum has today been sent to Bristol Asylum.

The Bristol patients were distributed to Asylums in Dorset, Wiltshire, Somerset (Wells), Somerset (Cotford), Devon, Exeter, Plymouth and Cornwall. The 1915 Annual Report of the Cornwall Lunatic Asylum reported the reception of 100 men and over 150 women from Fishponds Hospital.

Initially 520 beds were allocated to the War Office as Bristol's share of required hospital beds. The first contribution of 260 came from the Bristol Royal Infirmary, Southmead offered a like number in its newly built Infirmary Wards. As casualties mounted these had to be added to time after time The 1,460 beds in the Beaufort Hospital were by far the largest single contribution. In an emergency this could be increased by a further 180 patients accommodated on the floor.

Considerable alterations were necessary to equip the Asylum as a Military Hospital. This work was carried out at the War Office's expense and the hospital was designated the "Beaufort War Hospital, for the general medical and surgical treatment of sick and wounded soldiers."

The Asylum medical superintendent, Dr J.V. Blatchford became Colonel (RAMC) in Charge supported by his deputy Dr Philips in appropriate rank.

The Nursing Staff all female as was the custom at that time was provided by generally trained ladies of the Queen Alexander's Imperial Military Nursing Order colloquially called the Q.A's .

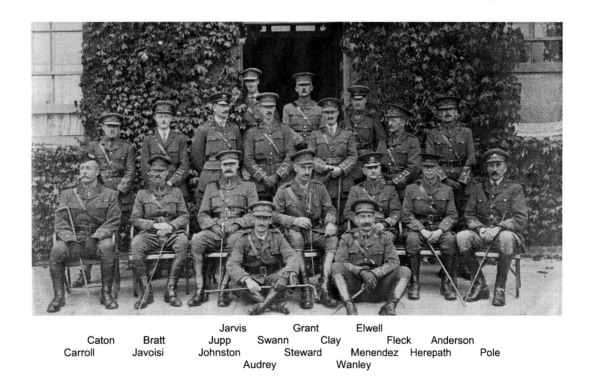

		Jarvis		Grant		Elwell		
	Caton	Bratt	Jupp	Swann		Clay	Fleck	Anderson
	Carroll	Javoisi	Johnston		Steward	Menendez	Herepath	Pole
			Audrey		Wanley			

Figure 25 Medical Staff 1915

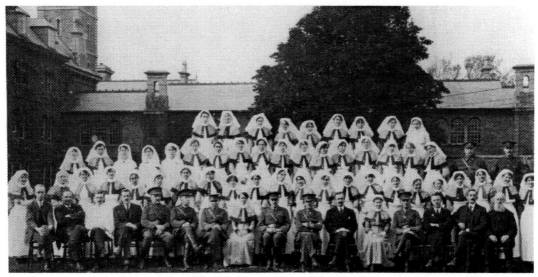

Dr Fleck is in front row 5th from left, and Dr Blatchford 7th from right.

Figure 26 Nursing, Medical and Administrative Staff

The mentally trained asylum attendants who had not been called up for military service were retained as orderlies and worked under the authority of the Q.A's.

The female mentally trained asylum nurses who had no general nursing qualifications served as auxiliary nurses and were also supervised by the Q.A's. This situation must have given rise to difficulties. The Asylum Matron was in charge of the laundry and in 1919 again took over authority for all the female beds in the hospital. No photograph has been found of this important staff group.

There is no record of the 45 men patients who were retained for work on the grounds and in the hospital departments and shops. Little information survives of their life.

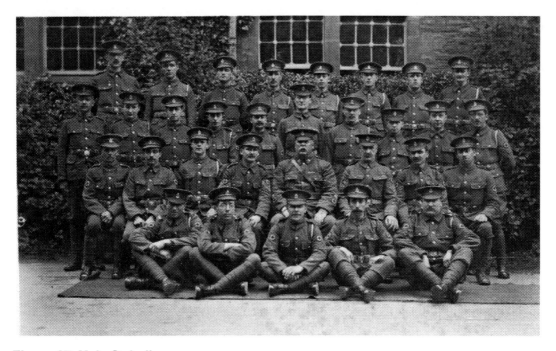

Figure 27 Male Orderlies

There are more photographs of the soldiers who were patients than the helpers, as enterprising photographers went around photographing many of the patients on the wards, giving us a record of the appearance of many of the wards. These are the only series of photographs of the inmates of the hospital that was made for public sale. In the days as an asylum this was forbidden.

One person who was aware of the existence of the helpers and of some of their problems was one of the early recruits to the nursing staff (RAMC), the artist Stanley Spencer, who joined up in July 1915. His paintings and writings give an insight into what the Hospital routine was like. He experienced little of the life of these 45 men with mental illness who remained behind in the hospital "to carry out menial tasks." He describes a patient who worked in the Head Male Attendants Office as

> one of the male 'loonies' known as 'Deborah' who acted as the Chief Male Nurse's orderly or runner." His face was long and egg-shaped with a short scrubby white beard and bald head. I felt he could claim some mystical discipleship with the Sergeant Major. If The Sergeant Major was God, Deborah was St. Peter. He slunk about with short shuffling steps and never looked up. If he did, it was only when he thought no one was looking. [1]

Another time he wrote "If I was like Deborah, the lunatic who doesn't know there is a war on. His sullen face and shifty eyes. I envied him the agony of being cut off completely from my soul."

Spencer described how one of the patients went berserk:

> I always get the feeling of a man possessed by devils when I see a man in a mad fit. I remember one man, he was perfectly all right, and then suddenly he was cast down and it took about 10 men to hold him. He was put into … a padded cell at first but that was not big enough to hold him so they spread 12 mattresses on the floor of a room and put him in there. There he raved for a day and a night and spat at everybody especially when he was being fed. The Sister used to hold his food to his mouth while two or three men held his arms down. His face gave me the feeling that he wanted to pray that the devil would come out of him. He was taken away but is now all right, in his right mind. Working like this is shocking but to know a man and like him and to know that man is going mad is awful. [2]

There were many aspects of life as an Army medical orderly of which he was critical. Ken Pople records that he suffered experiences in Fishponds "which almost stifled creative imagination", that in general he was not interested in recording the activities of the hospital, that he accepted the disciplines and routine of hospital life, "plenty to eat and staff quite reasonable" but that he found the place itself "damnably smug and settled down" and yearned for the activity of a non-medical regiment. On the other hand according to his brother-in-law Andrew Causey[3] he was enormously stimulated by his war experiences at the Beaufort Hospital; "He liked to distinguish between places where he had happy feelings and those where he had not; Bristol and Macedonia were among the former."

In a letter to James Wood, a fellow recruit stationed at Trowbridge Spencer wrote "I am thinking about the Beaufort War Hospital which the more I think about it, the more it inspires me. I think there is something wonderful in hospital life, 'doing things' is wonderful."

His hospital experiences had a profound effect upon Spencer. In his great work, the Oratory of All Souls, Sandham Memorial Chapel at Burghclere, the wall paintings made between 1926 and 1932 depict some aspect of his experiences during the Great War. Seven of the eight predella scenes are based on his recollections of the Beaufort War Hospital, as are the

[1] Royal Academy of Arts Catalogue 1980
[2] letter to Reverats from Spencer on 12th June 1916 (in Ken Pople. *A Biography of Stanley Spencer* 1991
[3] Andrew Causey in Royal Academy of Arts Catalogue 1908. Published in association with Widenfield and Nicolson, London

first and second paintings in the upper register. They are beautifully reproduced and described in the National Trust Booklet "Stanley Spencer at Burghclere." As he completed each painting, he arranged them around the walls. It is apparent that at first hospital scenes but then Macedonian subjects predominated and were awarded more prominent positions.

This church was dedicated, as the Oratory of All Souls on 25th March 1927. By this time two canvases were already completed. The first canvas in the series, (1927), was an idea derived from Beaufort Hospital. *Scrubbing the Floor* showed an orderly lying full length on the floor (said to be a patient, but possibly Spencer) with arms stretched forward whilst other orderlies approached with trays. He said that the corridor he based this on had windows in, but he omitted these. This predella is placed below the first painting after the Church building was completed in May 1927 which was, *The Arrival of a Convoy at the Hospital Gates* which was destined for the first arched space. At the time of painting the picture Spencer could not remember what the roadway looked like because at the time he was terrified of the lodge keeper whom he feared might pull him in for some minor disciplinary offence. He painted the road lined with rhododendrons. He later recalled that the gate was "a vile cast iron structure" and its keeper a fellow whom he "could imagine cutting my head off as easily as imagined him cutting off chunks of meat."

The next Beaufort painting to be completed (1927) was *Sorting and Moving Kit Bags*. The patients who were not bed-cases would point out their bags and the orderlies would then carry them to wherever the patient wanted them. This predella was placed underneath *Ablutions*. *Ablutions* has sinks that are very reminiscent of those in the mental hospital. In The National Trust booklet Duncan Robinson writes of the painting; "Spencer regarded the mundane activities of the hospital with a sense of religious ritual and the hospital pictures symbolise a quotation from St.Augustine's Impressions "ever busy yet ever at rest gathering yet never needing; guarding; creating; nourishing; perfecting."

The next picture in the registry is *Sorting the Laundry*. The Matron of the Asylum was in charge of the laundry. This may explain the lighter emotional atmosphere portrayed in this painting since she was not trained in the more formidable authoritarian manners of the Army nurses. Some of the workers portrayed are probably asylum patients, possibly all of them.

"Filling Tea Urns has as its theme the mystery of the everyday life of the mental patients who were confined to a separate wing of the hospital. They were only seen in the kitchens when orderlies and inmates collected tea urns for their respective wards from opposite sides of a Counter. He saw the inmate who stood with his urn on the far side of the room every day for a year without discovering who he was, or what lay down the passage into which he disappeared."

Frostbite may not appear to be related to Beaufort, but it was Spencer's job to scrape the patient's feet, a task of religious significance to him. The wall paper is sad to be that of a day room in the hospital.

Bedmaking is said to derive from a hospital ward in a requisitioned house in Salonika. The turned legs of the low bed however suggest the "epileptic" bed of the Bristol Hospital. One remains in the Museum.

Washing Lockers These large baths continued in use in the Bristol Mental Hospital into the 1930's and beyond. Spencer is said to have hidden between them.

Tea in the Ward. Duncan Robinson says that there is a story that, after his identity became known to the Matron at Beaufort, there was always more bread and jam on Spencer's ward, as this was the artists favourite diet.

That Macedonian subjects have later been given the more prominent places in Burghclere is a situation of demotion to which asylums became accustomed even when war converted them into more glamorous surgical functions as in the Beaufort. Pople, however, sweetens the pill when he concludes that, "no such prosaic institution as Fishponds Hospital could ever have had a more glorious memorial. Yet in one way the hospital deserved its accolade. Of the 29,434 patients who had been admitted in the 4 years of its existence only 164 had been lost in death, and of these were 30 civilian emergencies who had been rushed there during the influenza epidemic of 1918. The dedicated men and women who worked there, whatever their grumbles, served better perhaps than they knew."

In 1919 the army left the Beaufort and everything returned to normal, the same medical and administrative hierarchy, the same nursing staff less those who had been killed, the same patients returned from Gloucester, Somerset, Devon. From Cornwall they returned in three groups, the first seen off by the Visitors at 10am, 7th December 1919 "well dressed and well clad for the journey." Further groups departed on October 1st 1920 and October 13th 1920.

The first civilian patient was admitted on December 18th 1919.

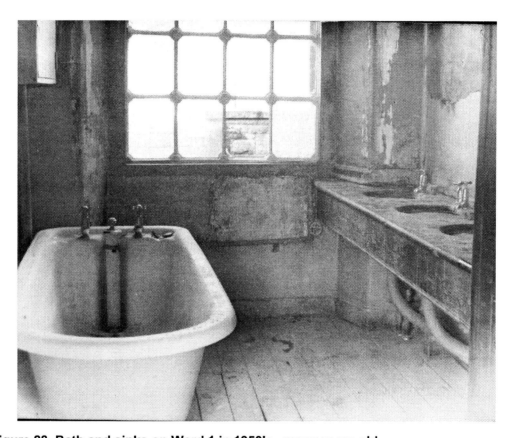

Figure 28 Bath and sinks on Ward 1 in 1950's - many years old

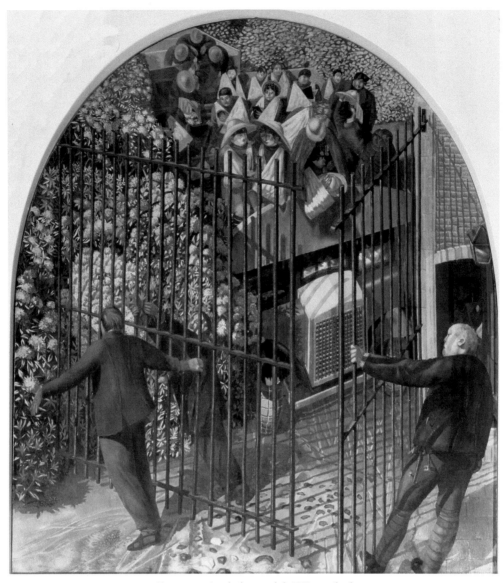

Convoy Arriving with Wounded

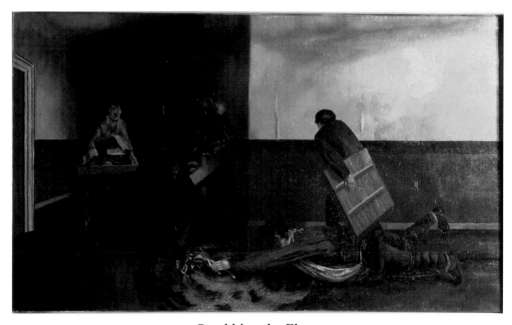

Scrubbing the Floor

PLATE 1

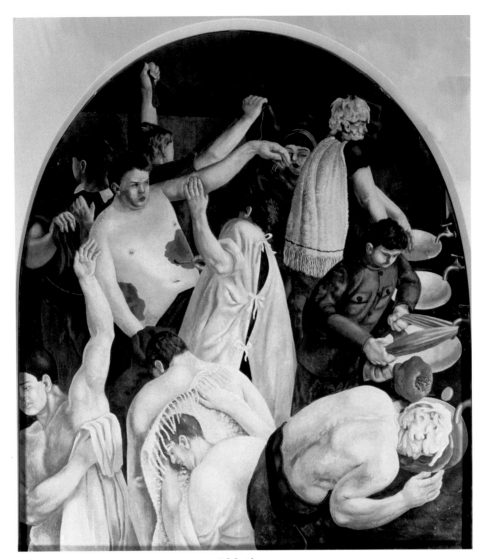

Ablutions

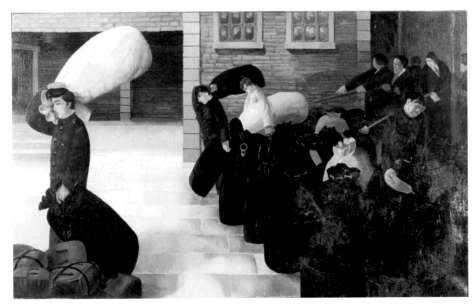

Sorting and Moving Kit-Bags

PLATE 2

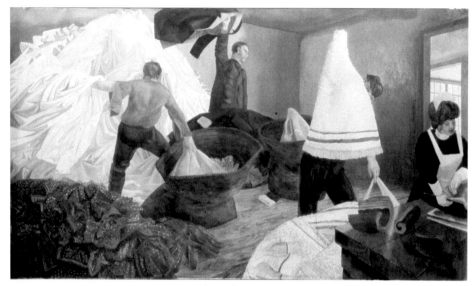

Sorting the Laundry

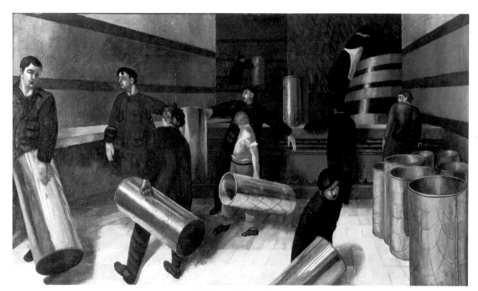

Filling Tea Urns

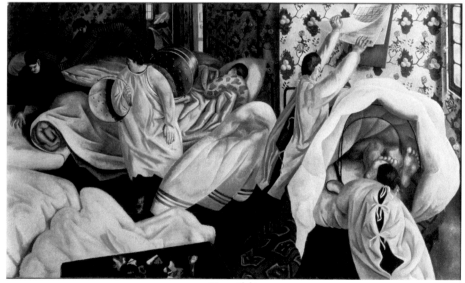

Frostbite

PLATE 3

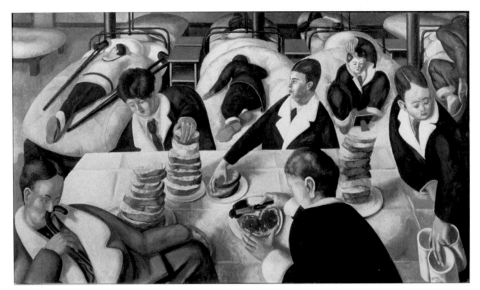

Tea in the Hospital Ward

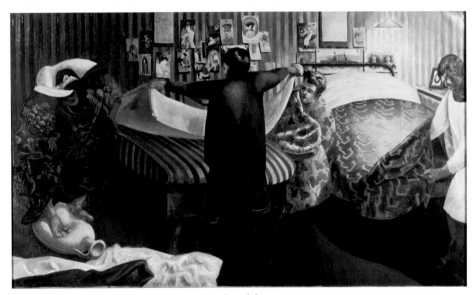

Bedmaking

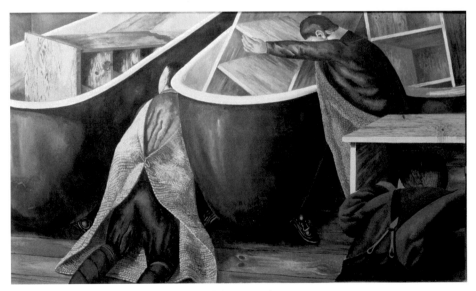

Washing Lockers

PLATE 4

From Asylum to Hospital 1919– 1936

The changes which followed the Armistice of 1918 were scarcely felt in the Bristol Lunatic Asylum, which returned to its pre-war name and traditions with its pre-war Visiting Committee and its pre-war medical superintendent who had been Colonel in charge of the Beaufort during the War. The last of the soldiers left on the 28th February 1919. Renovations started in May 1919. The first patients returned in September 1919.

The Board of Control referred to "the tasteful and apparently economical repair of the wards." A Commissioner, visiting on his own on August 12th 1920, referred to the interval since 1914, the last inspection, as "an important break in the continuity of history" and congratulated the Chairman, Alderman Pearson and the other members of the Committee of Visitors who had lent to the Army Council the institution with the whole of its staff and equipment, for use as a general medical and surgical hospital for sick and wounded soldiers. He paid tribute to the officers and staff of the Asylum for the admirable manner in which they carried out their orders and largely novel duties in the Beaufort Hospital.

Indeed, there they were again. The Chairman had become an Alderman and was supported by his old Vice-Chairman and by five of their pre-war Committee members. Col. Blatchford resumed as Dr Blatchford, Medical Superintendent with Dr Phillips his deputy, Rev James Fountaine, Chaplain and Arthur Orme, Clerk and Steward. By December 1920, 766 boarded out patients had returned. The appearance that nothing had changed was supported by the absence of any mention of the war in the Chairman's short report. Likewise the Chaplain's message came in two bland sentences which constituted his penultimate annual report. Dr Blatchford, proceeded as before, giving a routine summary of patient statistics and acknowledging the Commissioner's visit, reporting dances and other entertainment, expressing satisfaction about the produce of the farm and garden, assuring the Committee that the pigs made a considerable contribution to patients' diet and made a good profit, mentioning the artisan staff in a sentence of two lines, the nursing staff in four, the medical

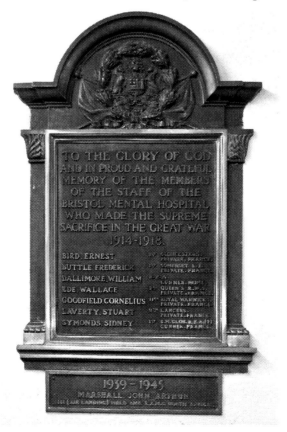

Figure 29 The Memorial to the Staff killed in both Wars. Now in Museum

in five. In three lines he proffered thanks to all, without any indication of the awful years which had led to the deaths of 7 male staff and unprecedented sufferings to patients and staff alike. No mention was made of the forty-five patients who remained behind in 1915 to work for the War Office in the hospital maintenance departments.

Little if anything had changed since pre-war. The hospital routine was spartan for staff and patients. Tom Long joined the nursing staff on 13th October 1919 following his army service. In 1950, he described the working conditions which he endured.

CITY & COUNTY ASYLUM
FISHPONDS, BRISTOL,

13.10. 1919

To *Thomas L Long*

I have to inform you that you are engaged as *Male nurse* in this Asylum on probation, at the expiration of which period you may leave if you do not like the duties, or your services may be dispensed with if you are found to be unsuitable. During the period of probation your engagement may be determined at any time without notice, and you are during the same period at liberty to leave at any time. After confirmation of your appointment by the Committee you will be expected to give and will receive a month's notice before leaving, except in the event of your breaking the Asylum Rules, when you will render yourself liable to instant dismissal, and forfeit all wages due ; but should you desire to leave without giving notice, you will be required to pay a sum of money equal to one month's wages. The salary you will receive at first will be at the rate of £ *2-0-0* per ~~annum~~ *week*, in addition to which you will be allowed ~~board (except bread) lodging, washing, and~~ uniform clothing. ~~During your service in the Asylum, 14 days' wages will be kept in hand by the Clerk.~~ *Board lodging + washing will be provided at a charge of 16/- per week.* This engagement is made subject to the provisions of the Asylum Officers' Superannuation Act, 1909.

You will be good enough to report yourself by entering on duty on *Monday* the *20th* day of *October*. next, and your doing so will be accepted as proof of your agreeing to the terms named above.

Yours, &c.,

J. V. Blackford

Medical Superintendent.

NOTE.—Uniform clothing is given to men after three months' satisfactory service, but should the uniform be withheld for any reason, no pecuniary allowance will be made.

Figure 30 Appointment letter for Thomas Long

The year 1921 dawned with a new stopgap Chairman, Alderman John Boyd. His predecessor George Pearson had retired on grounds of ill health. Having served for 32 years as a visitor, 22 of these as Chairman, he died in 1922. Alderman Boyd signed his Annual report on 31st March 1922 not as Chairman of the Lunatic Asylum but as Chairman of the Visiting Committee of the Mental Hospital for the City and County of Bristol.

One major advance in 1921 was the appointment of Mrs L M Pheysey to the Visiting Committee, the first woman so appointed. After 41 years the padre Rev James Fountaine, died and was not immediately replaced.

The hospital costs were rising. The total annual expenditure went from £29,128.00 in 1914 to £57,151.00 in 1920 and the maintenance rate rose from 10/6d [52.5p] to £1:11:0d [£1.55p] per patient per week. The Commissioners expressed disquiet that little of the increased maintenance costs was reflected in any improved benefits to patients citing the monotonous breakfast of bread and margarine and the long interval between tea and breakfast. The criticism was noted and next year the patients had a greater variety of foods with their evening meal, cake three days per week, jam twice weekly and strawberries occasionally.

Three Club wards were established for the ladies and there were two open wards on the men's side. They were described as very successful (1923).

An out-patient service was established in Bristol General Hospital. There was no pressure on admissions. Dr Blatchford showed his displeasure at the prevailing admission policy by recommending that epileptic patients would be better dealt with in a community which looked after such patients only. Otherwise he produced his usual report. He recorded in 1922 that the maintenance rate had fallen by 19/6 [97.5p] per week to 21/10 [£1.09p]. He reported the usual entertainments and dances, the provision of all necessary vegetables supplied to the hospital, a liberal supply of pork from the piggeries, of ward decoration and painting, staff pensions, the new Chaplain's arrangement of organ recitals and special soloists and of medical staff changes.

He retired on 2nd February 1924. In May the Commissioners recalled that he had held the office since 1904 and that during the War he was Superintendent and Medical Director of the Beaufort War Hospital. They praised him for his support and stimulation of outdoor activities particularly cricket. (Folklore says that he asked that his ashes be strewn on the hospital cricket pitch.) They commended him for his great interest in the scientific side of mental disorders and neurological problems but in spite of their laudations, they recommended better facilities for pathological and bacteriological examinations describing the existing accommodation as insufficient and the equipment as meagre. A better laboratory and a whole-time assistant was recommended "because" they said "no institution of such importance as this hospital should be without ample provision for the microscopic examination of post-mortem tissues, blood analysis, the bacteriological study of disease and the routine examination of milk and other foods."

This is how things stood in February 1924 but they were about to alter.

On March 10th 1924, Dr E Barton-White from the Dorset County Mental Hospital took up his appointment as Medical Superintendent. He immediately gave notice in a firm, quiet way that change was intended. He set about equipping a new research laboratory. Dr Hadfield, Specialist Pathologist, Bristol General Hospital was appointed to visit the hospital weekly to initiate and supervise the lab work. Under his influence a Chief Technician, Gilbert Pope, was appointed whom he trained to provide a day-to-day pathology service.

In 1928 Dr Hadfield was appointed Professor of Pathology in the London Hospital. He was succeeded by Dr A.L.Taylor who continued in the post until the inception of the National Health Service (N.H.S.) 1948.

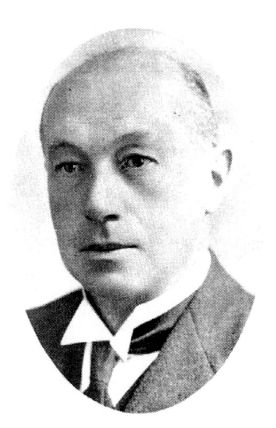

Figure 31 Dr Edward Barton-White Medical Superintendent 1924 - 1936

The lab was capable of routine examinations and of original research entailing histological tissue examination of organs including endocrine glands. In Dr White's time, many articles were published in the medical press and research results were presented e.g. to the Annual Spring meeting of the Royal Medico Psychological Association (R.M.P.A.)held in Fishponds on 10th February 1928 and at the South West Divisional Meeting of the R.M.P.A on 16th October 1928.

From 1925 onward, the annual Pathological Laboratory Report constituted an important and lively addition to the record of hospital clinical activity. Under the routine direction of the Gilbert Pope, it retained an influence through fair and foul days until its management was taken over by Frenchay General Hospital in the NHS reorganisation of 1974.

Under General Hospital Management the on-site path service was whittled down to a urine-testing and blood cell counting service and eventually removed to the site of Frenchay General Hospital. Glenside staff found the new service sluggish and at times reluctant. Few considered that the new service equalled that which it replaced.

The Commissioners of the Board of Control in their 1925 report said that they were satisfied that Dr Barton-White was keenly alive to the necessity of a certain amount of re-organisation to meet modern medical requirements. They probably underestimated what was happening. In his first year he hastened slowly. There was no overcrowding and so no problems in the much higher number of senile and hopeless cases admitted. Probably because of the manageable bed situation, the hospital was able to contain a recurrence of Dysentery but, in 1926, a further outbreak affected 49 men and 47 women and resulted in 3 deaths. The organism (flexner strain, see page 51) was then isolated and tested against standard strains by Professor Ledingham of the Lister Institute in London. The possibility of the immunisation of patients against this hospital strain was considered not to be worthwhile at that time. Later when the gross overcrowding recurred and when the spread of the infection could not be contained, a hospital vaccine was developed and routine inoculation of all new admissions with this vaccine continued until the fifties. The work on these organisms was carried out by Gilbert Pope.

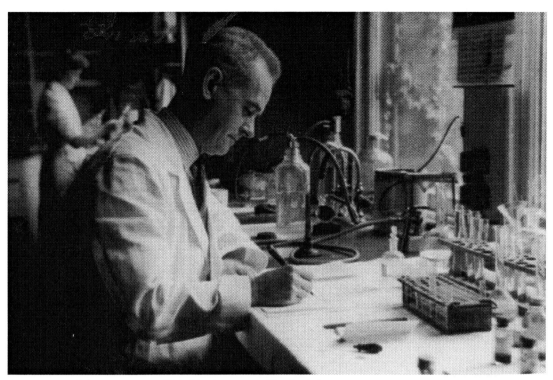

Figure 32 Gilbert Pope, Chief Laboratory Technician

Dr Barton-White provided an Out patient service in the Bristol General Hospital and in 1925 was appointed Lecturer in Mental Disorders in the University of Bristol. The clinical work in Fishponds was supported by a lengthening list of consultants in pathology, surgery, gynaecology, ophthalmology and in medicine by Dr Carey Coombs. More complete notes were made on admission, routine special tests were readily available. Attempts were made to assign the principal contributory causes to presenting clinical conditions but these had a limited horizon eg. insane heredity, alcohol, syphilis and general stress. By 1926 the changes in hospital activity were so noteworthy that the Commissioners praised the standard of professional work especially the character of clinical records and of autopsy examinations.

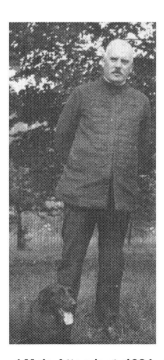

Figure 33 Charles Humber, Head Male Attendant 1924 - 1935

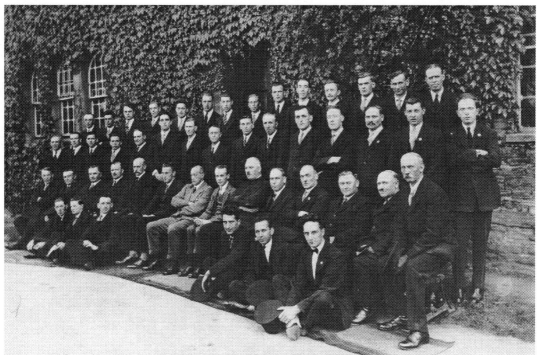

Bob Lerway; R.Baylis; F.Knight; ?A.H.Baldwin; Idris Williams; Tom Jones (farmer); →
Cecil Crowe;(?);(?); A. Redmond; Geo. Alfred Price; Cliff Veale; Tom Long; O.Grffiths
Dowling; (?); Tom Hollow; Jack Harrison; Henry Holmyard; Bob Hewitt; (?); Sam Upward; →
Tom Jones (Whippet); Geo. Beese; (?); (?); Fred Clifford; Bill Clutterbuck; (?)
J.Green; T.Rowan; Bill Vardy; Alf Pike; Geo.Jones; Dr Gordon Tresidder; Dr Barton-White; Dr.H.Smith; →
S.Charles Humber; George Whitehouse; Bill Jackson; Jack O'Connor; Henry Allen; Fred Moss
Cliff Lerway; George Pedley; Murphy;　　　Thomas; Hy Harrison; Emlyn Davies

Figure 34 Dr Barton-White, his Assistant I.T.O.'s and Male Staff

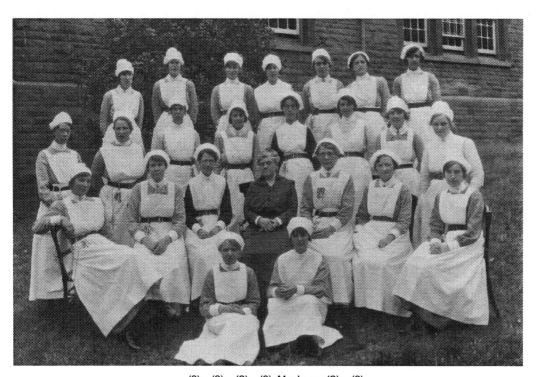

(?)　(?)　(?)　(?) Mrs Long; (?)　(?)
(?)　(?)　(?)　(?)　(?)　(?) Gilmour; Richards
(?)　M Parsons; C Cox (Deputy Matron); Miss Dunne (Matron); M Watkins; (?) (?)
(?)　　(?)

Figure 35 Nursing Staff

The nursing situation was unstable. In June 1924, three months after his own appointment, Dr White expressed his satisfaction at the appointment of a well trained Head Male Attendant, Charles Humber. Under his management, the male nursing staff was described as efficient and stable in their employment.

The same could not be said for the female department. There were then only 3 ladies with the certificate of the Medico Psychological Association (M.P.A.) Junior female staff usually left the service without obtaining a professional qualification. In 1925 Miss M.P.Dunn MBE, Matron retired after 27 years service.

She was replaced by Miss Dorothy Jones, the Deputy Matron. She was a young active woman who succeeded in turning round a near – catastrophic situation where there was "a continued lack of interest among the juniors." She had a special interest in and commitment to training. Lectures and Demonstrations by Medical Officers, by the Matron and by the Head Male Attendant were organised for junior nurses. The hospital was recognised as a training school and by 1927, 5 male and 7 female probationers passed the (now) Royal Medico-Psychological Association (R.M.P.A.) preliminary examination and 8 passed the final. In 1929 a Home Sister/Tutor was appointed, nursing recruitment improved and the turnover lessened. All Ward Sisters (13) and Charge Nurses (10) and their Deputies held the Certificate of the R.M.P.A. A forty-eight hour week was established. Lack of residential accommodation was identified as one of the main problems in keeping nurses after qualification and discussions with the Officers and Committee were held to seek a solution to this problem. A Nurses Home was built and occupied before Miss Jones' retired on her marriage in 1931. 'Twere better if she had waited just a slightly longer time to wed.

Staff shortage was made much more obvious by the re-appearance of the old demon of patient overcrowding. In 1925 there were 836 in-patients in the hospital, which figure had risen to 1024 in 1927 when the beds on the female side of the hospital were 24 over complement. Beds in the non-observation wards were often available but acute beds, infirmary beds and single rooms were usually occupied.

Although largely self-supporting the little supervision necessary for the Three Club wards established in 1922, could not be provided and they had to be closed.

Nevertheless small but significant improvements continued, eg. newspapers and books from the Red Cross and from other services were freely circulated in the wards, many patients had the freedom of the grounds and parole outside hospital was common, with relatives or with off duty staff. Dances and concerts were held weekly, and in 1926 a cinematic apparatus was placed in one of the large halls.
The practise of rewarding working patients with tobacco or other goods was replaced in 1926 by a tally system. In 1928 this was reported to be working well with 190 men and 150 women "paid" with tokens of 6d, 4d, 3d, 1½ d and 1d which could be exchanged in the canteen for articles of one's own choice. Thus it was hoped that more men and women would be persuaded to occupy themselves usefully.

Up to the 1930's there were few physical treatments available for mental illness apart for those employed for symptomatic relief.

Malarial treatment which was introduced by Wagner-Jauregg in Vienna in 1917 for General Paralysis of the Insane (G.P.I) was first used in Fishponds in 1927. Two male patients were infected with malaria, one of whom recovered sufficiently to be discharged. The other underwent the inevitable fate of the untreated case, physical and mental deterioration and death. A permanently mosquito proofed room was arranged in the male side of the hospital. If the treatment took place on a female ward, between May and October temporary mosquito proofing was required. The treatment continued to be used until the introduction of Penicillin in the 1940's. A six year survey from, 1931 to 1936, showed 72 cases treated of which 43 recovered sufficiently to be discharged from hospital, an impressive 60% recovery rate for an illness 100% fatal in pre-treatment days.

General Paralysis (or Paresis) of the insane is now uncommon. It is a tertiary manifestation of syphilitic infection occurring sometimes many years after primary infection in untreated or unsuccessfully treated cases. Before the introduction of malarial treatment it was invariably fatal within 2-3 years. Antibiotic treatment of syphilis in its early stages, has caused this once common disease to become a rarity.

In 1929 the Royal Commission on Mental Disorders let it be known that it was recommending that patients should be received into mental hospitals as voluntary patients without the formality of a magistrates order i.e without "certification." The resulting bill received Royal approval in 1930 and the Mental Treatment Act (MTA) came into operation on January 1st 1931.

Later that year, in April 1931, Dr Barton-White was taken in by a sham doctor.

Most of these gentlemen confine their activities to medicine and surgery. William Cecil Faulkiner alias Dr Norman Nelson Kirkup was doubly successful in his impersonations, posing both as a doctor and as a clergyman. Faulkiner was born in Belfast. As a boy he ran away to sea. In 1914 he enlisted in the R.A.M.C. He married in 1922 but his wife divorced him. Posing as a doctor he subsequently married a widow and defrauded her of her life savings. For this he was sentenced to 18 months imprisonment in 1929 and on his release from prison in January 1931 he started up a medical practice in Exeter. He immediately proposed marriage to Miss Court, a school teacher, the daughter of a farmer from Clevedon in Somerset. His proposal was accepted by her and he obtained her father's consent. In April 1931 he was appointed as temporary Assistant Medical Officer at the Bristol Mental Hospital, Fishponds. He was well thought of medically. He professed also to be a Clerk of Holy Orders. He carried out services for the burial of the dead. He conducted marriages, one of these was in the hospital church, which service he undertook for the then matron, Miss Margaret Jones. In hospital circles the story gained ground that the "doctor" actually wed Miss Jones. Happily she escaped that misfortune.

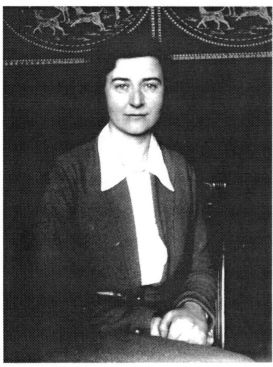
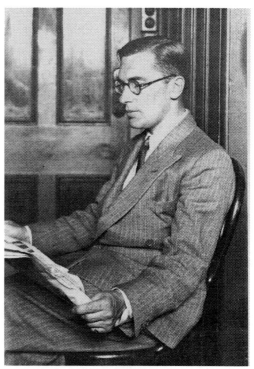

Figure 36 1932: Dr Penuel G. Grant   Dr Robert. E. Hemphill

From his safe haven in hospital he applied successfully for the position of surgeon to North Borneo Chartered Company. He presented testimonials covering 5 years during which time he claimed that he had been engaged by the American Church Missionary Society and by the Government Mental Health Authorities at Lucknow University. The job required that he be a married man so he borrowed £20 from Miss Court's father and he married her in October 1931. He borrowed a further £30 from her father for his passage to Singapore and £80 for his "wife's" return ticket. After they had sailed, it was discovered that he had been in communication with his lawful wife before he left England and during the voyage. Inspector Dunfield of the local Somerset Police Force travelled to Singapore to arrest him and to bring him home. He was tried for bigamy and for obtaining securities by false pretences. He was sentenced to 5 years penal servitude. Six months after his release from prison he continued his career as a doctor. At Liverpool quarter sessions in June 1938, his trial was described as "a chapter of the amazing life story of a most plausible liar." He pleaded that there must be something wrong with him that made him tell such deliberate lies and asked that he be prescribed treatment. The Recorder said: "I do not know whether yours is a case for mental treatment. The only treatment I can give you is 18 months with hard labour," which he thereupon dispensed. This was little benefit to Miss Jones.

Dr Barton-White pressed relentlessly for better conditions for staff and patients and this led to the provision of the new Nurses Home at Fishponds. He had been offered a temporary building but he eschewed any such solution. At the same time a house separate from the main hospital was built for the Medical Superintendent and married staff quarters were also provided.

He established the beginnings of a social work department with the appointment of the first hospital Welfare Worker, Miss D Bowen JP. She was assigned the duties of ascertaining patients' home conditions, of accompanying them where appropriate to Out-patients in Bristol General Hospital (B.G.H.) and of keeping in touch with them after discharge.

Miss Guyatt became matron in 1932.

The improvement in medical case records and the increase in the number of physical treatments for mental illness led to the appointment of two additional medical officers, Robert Hemphill and Penuel Grant, bringing the total doctor complement to five.

The Path Lab continued to provide professional interest and stimulation. In 1930 routine prophylaxis against the hospital strain of Flexner dysentery was introduced and became routine. Seven years later (1937) the procedure was commented on as having led to a complete absence of this infection for the previous two years. Inoculation against this disease on admission continued into the 1940's as did routine Wasserman Reaction until syphilitic infection became uncommon and G.P.I. rare.

Dr Barton-White hoped that pathological and psychological research could be centred in the University. Amongst the investigations he himself undertook was an examination into calcium metabolism in epilepsy. His clinical judgement mirrored current fashion when he reported that the newly installed X-ray department and dark-room would be used mainly in the diagnosis of tuberculosis but also "for the investigation of conditions of visceroptosis and intestinal stasis, frequent causes of melancholia and hypochondriasis."

He managed actively to maintain all his interests but toward the end of his service he became overburdened by planning and administration. His annual reports always comprehensive and forward-looking became more prosaic and less clinically exciting. From the late twenties he was concerned with the building of a new hospital. He was greatly disappointed when in 1928, negotiations broke down for the near-ideal site at Oldbury Court, Fishponds, a magnificent estate neighbouring Fishponds hospital. This was followed by further long negotiations. In 1930, the City Council purchased 260 acres of land for £24,300 in the Wild Country, (so named in the Ordinance Survey Map) Barrow Gurney, North Somerset. This was a difficult site, subject to flooding on the south side of Bristol 11 miles from Fishponds. Much of the planning of Barrow Hospital was placed on his shoulders.

He was concerned throughout by major national and local changes but he never lost sight of the "minor" alterations which underwrote these. He was concerned with patient and staff welfare, canteen and library facilities, radio, dances, concerts, washing facilities, diet. The patient's day was extended so that they could stay up later and listen to the evening radio. 'Talkies' finally arrived. A projector was bought for £353-4-0d in June 1933. It soon became an immediate major entertainment. The management of the Patients' canteen was placed on a more business-like footing and became the responsibility of the Clerk and Steward. A new automatic telephone system was installed at the cost of £537-7-6d.

He saw an improvement in the terms and conditions of nursing staff with the introduction of the 48 hour week. He oversaw the building of a Nurses Home at Fishponds and of accommodation for medical and other professional staff which the Commissioners said was "making capital progress." He established a welfare service department. The medical staff was well organised with active interest in clinical work and research. He established a strong team of visiting consultants.

He left a forward looking active hospital. Nurses had won the right to live out of hospital and succeeded in negotiating a living out allowance. The rapid change caused nervous strain; the Matron Miss Guyatt retired on medical grounds on 1st January 1935 and Charles Humber the Head Male Nurse was "forthwith pensioned" from Dec 1st 1935, and replaced by Mr Fred Foster. This may have had more to do with the fact that Miss Lyons, the new matron had been appointed in charge of all nursing staff, male and female, in the new hospital.
The new Fishponds nurses home opened in 1932. There were 95 R.M.P.A. trained nurses on the staff (60 male, 35 female) of whom 13 were male Charge Nurses and 11 were Ward Sisters. There were 140 (61male, 79 female) nurses on day duty and 28 (11 male, 17female) on nights. All under the leadership of a recently appointed Matron and a New Chief Male Nurse. The staff situation was at a peak.

The quality of patient life was improving steadily.

Dr Barton-White served as Medical Superintendent for twelve years. His 1935 annual published in March 1936, ran to 8½ pages, described a psychiatric regime changed beyond recognition since his appointment. He retired in October 1936, earlier than was expected. He left the presentation of the 1936 annual report to his successor Dr John Black-Martin.

The Start of Barrow Hospital - 1936– 1939

In October 1936 Dr J.J.B Martin of Dorchester was appointed Medical Superintendent. Although only 3 months in post, he presented the annual medical report of 1936 consisting of a record of hospital activity mainly under the regime of Dr White.

There was excitement in the air. The City Council had sanctioned £30,950 for the modernisation of engineering services, heating and hot water systems, kitchen, laundry and bake-house. An important scheme for general reconstruction and re-organisation of ward accommodation was being prepared, but towering over all these plans and proposals for Fishponds was the £39,285 which had been authorised as the first instalment of capital for the building of the new hospital - Barrow Hospital – the first phase of which was to provide accommodation for 395 patients.

In spite of its problems, Fishponds was clinically active. The admission rate had risen to 370 (164m, 206f), 34% of whom were on a voluntary basis, as allowed under the new 1930 voluntary treatment Act. The quality of life of patients was improving. Restraint was not employed and the use of padded rooms was reduced to a minimum. A second welfare worker was appointed. Social activities were interesting and varied. The Theatre Royal players entertained staff and patients, the staff band played fortnightly for dances. Ground parole was extended to 100 of 470 male in-patients and to 54 of 660 ladies. Profits from the canteen provided outings, a wireless in all the wards and books for the library.

As a result of the introduction of the forty-eight hour working week for nurses, there was an increase of 38 (14 men, 24 women) in the establishment. Many of these were trained in handicraft instruction so that the number of idle patients was declining, although this trend was restricted by a recurring difficulty in maintaining an adequate female nursing staff on the wards.

The Path Lab continued its active contribution. The hospital escaped an epidemic of Diphtheria early in the year, although it was not so fortunate later when the staff were affected by an epidemic of haemolytic streptococcal tonsillitis. There were no fatalities.
Amongst the patients 10 of the 133 male admissions and 6 of the 120 ladies returned a positive WR test for syphilis. Eleven of these suffered from General Paralysis of the Insane of whom 7 were treated with malaria. Four of them recovered, and were discharged 3 remained in hospital at the year's end, 2 of whom were improved.

Nothing unusual happened in 1937. Barrow Hospital was a-building and nearing completion and was the subject of much discussion. The capital building cost was high, approximately £900. per bed (the cost of a working man's house). It was going to be only one quarter built but it was calculated that when complete this figure would reduce to about £600 per bed. It was proposed that patient admission begin by Spring 1938.

It was decided that the entire nursing staff of the two hospitals male and female should be in the hands of Miss Lyons, the Matron stationed in Fishponds. There were 83 female nurse resignations during Miss Lyon's second year as Matron. Mr Fred Foster the new Head Male Nurse also resigned.

Overcrowding in Fishponds "again engaged the attention" of the Committee. An "important scheme for general reconstruction" to relieve some of the congestion on the female side of Fishponds hospital was introduced by the Chairman. A complete scheme for the modernisation of the heating and hot water supply, laundry apparatus and bake-house was approved by the Council but did not get off the ground.

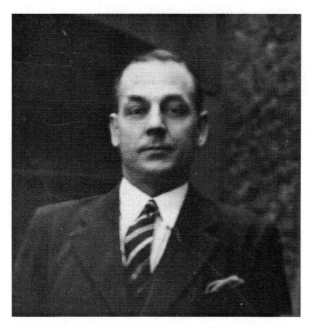

Figure 37 Fred Foster C.M.N. December '36 – December '37

Dr Martin produced an unremarkable second annual report with routine remarks about occupational therapy, welfare work (Miss Gillford was appointed as assistant), amusements, parole, and visits of inspection. Only Dr A. L. Taylor's report on Pathology Service retained its vitality. Dysentery prophylaxis with the hospital vaccine, again proved successful. During the 8 years after the introduction of preventative inoculation, 15 cases of Dysentery were notified compared with 157 during the previous 7 years. Dr Hemphill produced negative results in his enquiry into Calcium Blood Serum levels in Dementia Praecox and reported limited success in the treatment of noisy and restless patients with Sodium Amytal. Dr Barber continued his therapeutic trial of Prominal in epilepsy and demonstrated "remarkable improvement" in 8 of 11 patients treated during the year.

The maintenance rate went from 25/- (£1.25) per week to 28/- (£1.40) per week per patient. There were 348 admissions, 31% voluntary, bringing the resident total to 1,132. The Medical Superintendent criticised the continuing use of the Public Assistance Institution as an admission hospital owing to their arrangements over which the mental hospital had no control; he reiterated his preference for direct admissions. Transfer of chronically ill patients from Fishponds to Stapleton P.A.I. under Section 25 of the 1890 Lunacy Act averaged 46 per year for the previous 10 years. This ceased, so it was calculated that if Barrow attracted private and voluntary patients in large numbers, there would be overcrowding again in 5 years time after its occupation.

In February 1938 the Commissioners described the condition of Fishponds as "quiet" and ascribed this (amongst other reasons) to "the latitude allowed to patients, attention to recreation and amusements, well organised occupational therapy and the exceptionally good and generous dietary." They also noted that the clinical notes were well kept, that a loose leaf system with folders was being introduced and the notes were to be kept in clinical rooms on the wards. In fact it was nearly 10 years before clinical records reached the wards.

Alderman Mrs Pheysey who had been the first woman member of the Visiting Committee became Chairman in 1938. She was the first woman to occupy this position.

Although not officially opened until 3rd May 1939, Barrow Hospital received its first patients in May 1938. The Visiting Consultant staff was common to both hospitals, but a different approach was immediately apparent in the dissimilar titles accorded to the workaday medical staff. In Barrow the doctors were appointed as Senior Physician, Assistant Physician and Research Worker. In Fishponds the older appellation of Assistant Medical Officer applied.

Soon other inter-hospital difficulties were evident. Mrs Pheysey wrote "despite the transfer of nearly 300 patients, the rate of admissions continues to disappoint the hope that statutory beds in Fishponds may be reduced."

The high cost of maintenance in Barrow, 35/6d (£1.78) per patient per week, was explained by the larger number of staff required by smaller units and by new types of medical treatment, by increased administrative expenses and by addition of a large figure for inter-hospital transport. Dr Martin commented on the difficulty likely to be experienced by an executive officer retaining full control of two units separated by ten miles of busy traffic and he averred that "the inevitable tendency will be for Barrow and Fishponds to develop as separate and independent units."

In considering future developments, he criticised the lack of Local Authority development of mental health facilities in the City of Bristol. He questioned the statutory division of facilities for the treatment of mental diseases and mental deficiency, why some cases of mental disease should be afforded hospital treatment and others institutional facilities and why these services should be divided amongst different committees and authorities. He expressed the hope that "in the near future some effort is made to evolve a comprehensive scheme", to the benefit of individual patients and ultimately to the reduction of the residual chronic hospital population.

Neither in Barrow nor in Fishponds was there suitable accommodation for patients' occupation although the number of patients engaged in occupational therapy continued to rise. "Paradoxically" wrote Dr Martin "it is becoming increasingly difficult to find working patients necessary for the essential departments of the hospital." He ascribed this partly to the division of the hospital population between Barrow and Fishponds "and in part to the outlook of the patient (who) declares that he or she has come into hospital for treatment and not for work and it is not easy to persuade able bodied patients that work is a moral duty."

Whilst Barrow was being built, the upkeep of Fishponds was neglected. Dr Martin considered that it was "impossible to reconcile the modern wards at Barrow with the shabby and unsanitary wards at Fishponds and yet these are part and parcel of the same hospital and in theory at least, there should be frequent interchange of patients between the two places." The interior fabric of Fishponds was in need of repair, the entire water system required renewal and the electric wiring was old and faulty but the major reconstruction which had been planned would not now be carried out "in view of the large capital expense already incurred at Barrow." The necessary repairs, re-decoration and even minor sanitary and hygienic improvements remained undone and it was evident that there would be no reduction in the number of statutory beds.

Dr Martin was apprehensive about the dangerous concentration of patients in Fishponds. As war loomed he had the wards surveyed with a view to strengthening them and protecting them from bomb blast. The patients were drilled, gas masks were supplied, Air-raid precaution (A.R.P) lectures given to staff and the hospital fire brigade was re-organised.

By the end of 1938, it was known that Barrow would be evacuated in the event of war. Nevertheless it was officially opened by Sir Lawrence Brock, CBE Chairman of the Board of Control on May 3rd 1939.

Barrow was a considerable improvement over existing accommodation, as different in its way as Fishponds was from St Peters in 1861.

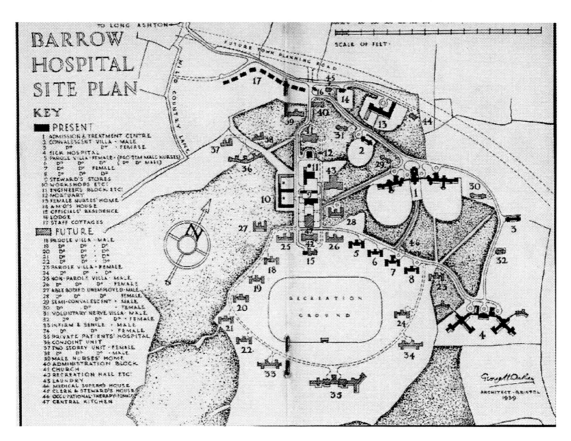

Figure 38 Barrow Hospital as planned

In his address at the opening Dr Barton-White described existing hospitals as built like barracks under one roof which though comfortable, provided little relief to those sensitive to their environment, with no adequate means for proper classification. Treatment in the hospitals like Fishponds which was similar to practically all the mental hospitals in the country was, he said, "well nigh impossible... and it became evident that hospitals built on the villa system breaking away from the institutional atmosphere provided all essentials for the realisation of satisfactory results where the environment is peaceful and conducive to rest and containment and where there is full scope for proper classification." He also expressed a less liberal but then not uncommon view, the result of which was soon to contribute to cataclysmic world disaster: "Though the goal we aim at is the prevention of disease, so long as man shows less consideration for the welfare of future generations of his own species than his care in breeding racehorses and pedigree dogs, we must be prepared to deal with the results and the large hospitals for the treatment of mental illness will remain a necessary charge upon us."

As advisory consultant to the Visitors, Dr Barton-White lauded the Architect, Sir George Oatley and the Commissioners of the Board of Control, Sir Hubert Bond and Mr John Kirklaw. He described the principles on which the hospital was based and expressed the view that administration in conjunction with Fishponds would lead to an "interchange of patients and of staff at any time." He did not comment on the fact that only one quarter of the total proposal had been completed but Sir George Oatley spoke of the unfinished business when he recorded that his plan catered for "an ultimate total of 1,150 patients" of which, 375 beds were presently commissioned including the Sick Hospital, the Admission and Treatment Centre. In fact no part of the remainder of the 1,150 projected beds was ever completed so that there was from the start an imbalance in the available types of accommodation. The benefits of classification were thus reduced.

One of the greatest practical problems in the new hospital was the installation of direct current electricity (DC) and which gave rise to continuing difficulties until the installation of alternating current (AC) in the fifties.

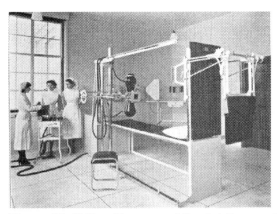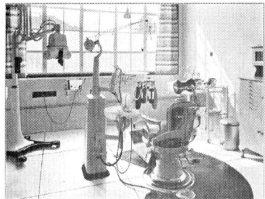

Figure 39 X-Ray Room and Dental Room at Barrow

During its first year of life, almost 50% of admissions to Barrow were on a voluntary basis. Physical standards within the hospital were excellent, but only private patients were allowed to wear their own clothes "because of storage problems."

The Admission Hospital had a treatment centre with rooms for massage, dental and ophthalmic treatment, physiotherapy and X-ray. The clinical records were kept on the wards each in a separate folder. The Pathology Laboratory was supervised by Dr A.L.Taylor of the Bristol General Hospital who continued the routines which he had established in Fishponds, where little pathology work was now done until Barrow closed again at the outbreak of war.

The medical staff, Gibson, Hemphill and Stengel was supported by a comprehensive panel of consultants. Hemphill and Stengel were active in research. Professor Golla and Mr Walter of the Burden Neurological Institute had access to all the laboratory and technical facilities and "co-operated very fully" in research and treatment.

Cardiazol convulsion therapy was introduced in 1937 and reported on by Hemphill, Gibson and Coates. Electro-convulsive treatment (ECT) was first used in 1939. Its complete loss of memory of the time immediately before and after treatment, was much less distressing to the patients but Cardiazol was considered to be clinically more effective by staff. Throughout 1939 and 1940 Professor Golla and Mr Grey Walter visited the hospital several times weekly to carry out the treatment using the Ediswan machine they had designed. Of the first thirty-seven patients treated with ECT, thirteen were reported to have recovered and eleven to have improved. E.C.T. was "extended to schizophrenics and manic-depressive cases." Of the first 75 female patients treated 20 recovered, 22 improved and 33 failed to benefit. Improvement was marked and most consistent in cases of agitated melancholia. An example of the Ediswan 'Electro-convulsere Therapy Apparatus' used in the Hospital can be seen at the Hospital Museum.

Little or no progress was made toward inter-hospital co-ordination and gaps in the levels of care and treatment were evident. At Fishponds heating and hot water services were causing "considerable disorganisation." This in turn caused all other activity to be postponed. In fact the only progress consisted of preparations for war. The cellars and wards were strengthened and protected against bomb blast, the patients being drilled and issued with gas masks.

In June 1939 there were 1,287 patients in residence, 292 in Barrow, 33 in Grove Road and 962 in Fishponds. Grove Road was closed.

On September 2nd 1939 the day before war broke out, these patients in need of continuing treatment were transferred to Fishponds. On September 3rd, war was declared and the Royal Navy took over Barrow resulting in a loss to the Bristol Mental Health Services of 375beds and increasing the grave overcrowding in Fishponds. In spite of having fallen into disrepair the house at 12 Grove Road, Redland which had been closed in 1938 was reopened for the reception of 30 female patients.

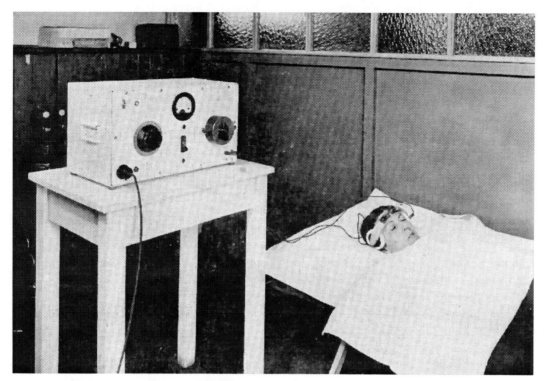

Figure 40 The Ediswan E.C.T. Apparatus

The War Years: 1939 - 1945

In October 1939 Alderman Mrs Pheysey resigned as Chairman of the Visiting Committee and Alderman Wise took over. In his first annual report, whilst acknowledging the overcrowding of accommodation and the shortage of staff he described the hospital as "efficiently managed and the buildings in good repair."

Those patients unfit for discharge had returned from Barrow to Fishponds. The number of admissions during the year was 411 the highest on record to date, the average number resident was 1,236. Dysentery which had been absent from the hospital for seven years broke out in September caused by the same organism (B-Flexner Z-X) which caused previous epidemics.

Dr Martin referred to "another violent transition" in the management of the hospital and complained that his task was becoming increasingly difficult. He reported that social life was going on much as usual except that special concerts and entertainment's were less frequent. He expressed concern about the dangerous state of installations and equipment. Many wards were still unheated and he complained that "it has been discovered rather late in the day that the water supply is deficient." The return of patients to the squalor of Fishponds greatly raised his anxieties. As the war progressed he found it increasingly difficult to cope.

Shortages of staff got worse and worse. On the outbreak of war 10 male nurses including 2 senior officers joined the Services as did an assistant baker and an engineer's labourer. By the end of 1940, 42 members of the male staff were serving in the forces. Thirty-nine (39) out of 56 female nurses left the service within 2 months of joining. The remainder stayed, on average for 4 1/2 months. The Mental Nurses (Employment and Officials) Order 1941 came into operation in August 1941 and made it a punishable offence for mental nurses to leave their employment except under certain conditions. This was of limited benefit to the problem of recruitment. In 1939, 19 members of staff qualified as RMPA nurses. In 1940, 17 were successful and from then on during the war years fewer and fewer qualified.
Staffing difficulties affected all departments. The medical situation became very difficult. Initially Dr.Stengel continued his research but he left during 1940, thus bringing to a close his work on pre-senile dementia. He and Hemphill published a couple of papers. Hemphill also published with Grey Walter and with Max Reiss whose co-operation in endocrine research (which was to be so important later), was reported for the first time. Dr Gibson a young and active medical officer resigned and was replaced by an older, retired doctor.

The close relationship continued with the Burden Neurological Institute but the fees paid to Golla & Grey Walter for treating patients with psychotherapy were discontinued; it was considered that E.C.T. superseded this treatment.
Pre-frontal leucotomy operations were carried out in 1941- 1943 by Mr F. W. Willway and by Mr Lambert Rogers at the Burden Neurological Institute.

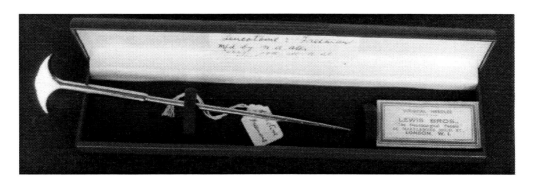

Figure 41 Freemans Leucotome (Chicago) used at the Burden Inst.

Max Reiss continued his research into endocrinological factors in psychiatric illness. The Burden staff was added to the list of honorary consultants to Fishponds hospital in recognition of the help which they offered in the dire staff situation which obtained in 1942/43

In spite of very difficult conditions an appearance of normality was sought and life was reported as progressing smoothly. A Report on Air Raid Precautions tells a contrary story. Since December 8th 1939, a Fire Watching patrol of the upper floor of the hospital was in operation and a minimum of 20 men were on call in the Hospital at night in addition to the Fire Brigade. A roof spotting scheme was instituted on July 1st 1940 when the equipment of a decontamination room was completed. The protection of ground floor windows and of skylights with wire-netting was carried out as materials became available. Disintegrating sandbags were replaced by brickwork and blast walls were erected to sub-divide the ground floor wards. Additional trap-doors were fixed in ceilings, air shafts were cut to give access to roof spaces and walking ways laid in the roof voids.
Bristol was the subject of severe enemy bombing. Fire-watchers on the flat-roofed administration building watched the City burn whilst high explosives burst all around and 'Purdown Percy', the anti-aircraft gun on the nearby Purdown hill was deafening in its barely reassuring cacophony.

The Medical Superintendent became more and more anxious and caused patients to be brought down to the basements when the air raid alert sounded. Morale was not improved by the nightly trudge to the cellars, which were lined with service pipes and gloomy in the extreme. They were not returned to their overcrowded ground floor wards until the all-clear was sounded, sometimes hours later. Dr Martin had the face of the tower clock painted black lest enemy bombers identify the white dial as a bombing target.

Dr Martin became increasingly apprehensive about the patients welfare. In November 1940 he went on sick leave. He had presided over the hospital during 5 exciting and difficult years. The opening of Barrow Hospital and 16 months later its closure gave too little time for the establishment of a settled routine and was accompanied by intra-professional conflicts. Its requisition by the Navy temporarily solved some of these problems but failed to find an answer to the unsolved question of how to deal equitably with "chronic" and "acute" psychiatric cases. The outbreak of World War II and the administration of a twelve hundred bedded hospital under fearful conditions accompanied by staff shortages placed severe strain on him. He retired on health grounds in 1941. He was succeeded in a substantive capacity by Dr Herbert Smith. His reports before he too retired, were more informative than those of his immediate predecessor and gave a clearer view of the social and medical difficulties that accompanied the fourth year of the war.

Forty-four staff members were now in the Forces. The Staff Comforts Fund Committee kept in postal contact with them and sent parcels. Jack Speed (Nursing Staff) was posted a POW in Germany. A letter was received in mid 1943 from Micheal O'Loughlin (Nursing Staff) who had previously been reported "missing" after the fall of Singapore. Gerry Dooley (Administrative Staff) previously "presumed dead" was officially reported a prisoner of war in Malaya.

Seventeen new nursing staff joined the hospital of who 10 left within the year. Twenty-two left the service overall. In spite of the current legal restraints, it was nearly impossible to retain suitable people.

The Auxiliary Fire Service (A.F.S.) had its headquarters in the hospital. The Fire Brigade and Fire Watchers together with other staff formed a Club "with the aim of organising and directing dances, indoor and outdoor games etc" which relieved the monotony of the watch.

The Canteen continued to supply extra comforts to patients and following the increase in duty on tobacco, the value of credit given to working patients was adjusted. The farm made money. Decorations, alterations and repairs were " on a much reduced scale."

When Dr Hemphill went down with phthisis in June1942 the Medical staffing was reduced to two working members. On return in November he was fit only for part-time duty. Dr.Collinson an elderly locum went sick and resigned his temporary appointment, Dr Kelly a temporary locum was suddenly taken ill and died the next day and Dr Gadeden a locum tenens appointed in July soon went ill and left in November. This left the medical cover of the hospital to Dr P G Grant and Dr H Smith. They received some help from Professor Golla, Dr Hutton and Mr Grey Walter of the Burden Neurological Institute. The Board of Control expressed surprise that the essential services of the hospital were working "so efficiently and so smoothly", and described it as very creditable that the newly introduced treatments were being carried on in spite of the shortage of nursing and medical staff. They cited ECT in agitated melancholia, hormone treatments, Epanutin in epilepsy and Derris root in scabies, all of which they said indicated the continuation of the tradition of research and the early introduction of new physical treatments.

After 19 years service Dr Herbert Smith retired on superannuation on May 1ˢᵗ 1944. Dr Robert Hemphill was appointed Acting Medical Superintendent.

Mr. I. J. Wise the Chairman wrote in the eighty-third Annual Hospital Report; "Your Committee have appointed Dr R.E. Hemphill, their Acting Deputy Medical Superintendent and Director of Clinical Services to be Medical Superintendent … Dr Hemphill has achieved a considerable reputation as a worker in the field of mental research and your Committee are confident that under his direction the Hospital will be kept well abreast of the changes which are foreshadowed in the post-war mental health services. In this connection your Committee desire to draw particular attention to the paragraph in the Medical Superintendent's report regarding out-patients in Bristol Royal Infirmary which represents a new departure." This refers to the closure of the Out-Patient Clinic at 12 Grove Road which Hemphill wrote

> … has been discontinued since April of this year (1944) when the Board of the Royal Hospitals placed me in charge of the newly formed Department of Psychiatry at the Bristol Royal Infirmary branch. This arrangement enables new patients to attend for diagnosis and to receive further advice or special treatment, if necessary... Attendances have increased considerably. Record keeping is facilitated and the desirable liaison between voluntary and mental hospital has been effected. Scope for teaching students has, of course, been increased.

Hemphill took over management of a hospital with wavering morale and a staff situation close to crisis point. The male nursing staff numbered a mere 60 for 522 patients whilst the female nursing staff stood at 56 where the pre-war number of 130, was itself inadequate. He himself had barely escaped from convalescent status but his drive and energy immediately became evident. Even the undertaking of mundane administrative mental hospital duties could not hide his enthusiasm for the newly formed Department of Psychiatry at the B.R.I. Out-patient attendance increased and a new phase in teaching began.

In May 1944, Dr. Penuel Grant was the only doctor in residence. In that month Dr. Robert Klein formerly Director of the Neurological Institute, Prague and I were appointed, bringing the number of working doctors to three. The average number of in-patients was 1217, an increase of 31 over 1943.

Hemphill's first annual report, written within one month of his appointment, contained no fireworks. He reported the use of Electro-shock Therapy in suitable out-patients where it had proved "extremely useful." There had been research into the role of endocrine glands in mental disorders and Max Reiss had "co-operated vigorously" in the work and in treatment. Dr Hutton of the Burden Neurological Institute had studied personality and other psychological changes in patients after Pre-frontal Leucotomy. Mr Willway had died. The inability to provide Leucotomy for patients in Fishponds was regarded as a deprivation. Hope was expressed that "with more surgical help this situation will improve."

In 1945, Penicillin was used for the first time in G.P.I. The mental condition of the patient improved but he unfortunately died of overwhelming complications – aortitis and pneumonia.

The absence of an Insulin Department was addressed. Miss Marsh, the Deputy Matron spent a fortnight in Crichton Royal Hospital Dumfries to study this treatment and I visited Warlingham Park Hospital, Croydon for the same purpose. Miss Diffley a doubly qualified nurse was appointed in nursing charge of a newly established Insulin department where treatment started early in 1945. In this treatment patients were put into an insulin-induced coma for a time. It was seen as an effective treatment.

In 1945 clinical tempo moved up several gears. The Chairman of the Visitors reported that he was particularly pleased to tell the members that a letter had been addressed to the Medical Superintendent by the Chairman of the Board of Control congratulating the medical and nursing staff on their work, which he considered to be a good augury for the future when Barrow Hospital would be available as an admission and treatment centre.
Dr Grant and I shared the routine hospital duties day and night, three 24 hour stints per week and every second weekend. Late in 1944, Dr Pearse O'Malley joined the staff. Later still as staff numbers grew duty rosters became less onerous.

Dr Grant had been appointed 12 years previously at the same time as Hemphill and spoke sympathetically of his idiosyncrasies. She was the doctor who had kept things ticking over. She explained the Medical Officer's routine responsibilities: three ward rounds per day, morning, lunch-time and night. Each patient to be examined on admission, then at least once every week for the month after admission and then monthly for the next eleven months. Thereafter twice per year, one of which examinations had to carry a statement of the patients physical health, - the annual "physicals" and "mentals." She knew the routines involved in relationships with the Board of Control. Reports to them were returned for modification, for every inaccuracy. She knew a great deal about the "workings" of the hospital. The re-organisation of 1948 and the bustle of the 50's unsettled her but she continued to work in a shy, retiring manner until retirement.

On May 4th 1944 in the Committee Room Dr Grant introduced, the new boys to Robert Hemphill, the Medical Superintendent. Klein and I took up duty as Assistant Medical Officers on the same day. Klein lived with his wife and son in a hospital flat. He took charge of the admission wards of the hospital. Dr Grant continued in charge of the female wards and I was responsible for the male wards.

Dr Grant next carried out the formal introductions to Henry Adams, the Hospital Engineer, then to Alfred Baldwin the Chief Male Nurse and to his deputy Cyril Bryant and to his Assistant Tom Hollow. Their welcome was authentic. In spite of their evident problems their morale was high and they obviously felt that whatever the new medical officers were like they were bound to be an improvement. They explained their current routines. Each day would start with a cup of tea and perusal of the mail. All outgoing mail had to be passed as inoffensive by the Nursing Officer and if in doubt letters were referred to the Medical Officer. Correspondence which was unacceptable was returned to the patient unless it was addressed to any one of the specified authorities. This was followed by discussion of hospital happenings of the previous day and the current day's requirements. A formal round of all the male wards then ensued accompanied by the senior nursing officer. The ward day and night reports, were examined, enquiry made into any untoward event so reported and discussion of current problems with the Charge Nurse on each ward. Much of the routine daily round was spent in the infirmary (MI) and convalescent (MC) wards. Sick patients were nursed on each of these. There were 12 wards on the male side - one of which was the Bungalow which was separated from the main building by a couple of hundred yards. It and the so called Work Ward were the only unlocked wards for men and between them housed 40 - 50 patients.

All routes of access into and out of the hospital grounds were closed. At 11pm the main gates were locked by the resident lodge porter, who was also the hospital telephonist and who then went off duty and was available only in emergency throughout the night. All wards and hospital doors were locked by night and all except three wards, two male and one female were locked 24 hours per day.

The black-out had made living conditions very uncomfortable. Many ground floor windows continued to be bricked up so that the grossly overcrowded wards were stuffy, particularly by night. The smell of over heated humanity, paraldehyde, cats urine, coffee and boiled cabbage is an odorous amalgam not easily forgotten.

In spite of the shortage of nursing staff – the men were in the Forces, the women were more than 50% below strength, the standard of care was good and the desire to learn was remarkable even amongst the older staff. Any offer to teach was eagerly accepted and clinical manoeuvres were willingly supported; the annual physical examinations of 500 patients were usually keenly observed by the nurses seeking instruction.

Gilbert Pope, at first the only and later Chief Lab technician was a man of resource and experience. He had been well trained by Dr A L Taylor, the Honorary Pathologist to the Bristol General Hospital and was capable of many complicated examinations. He carried out routine blood, urine, sputum and other investigations. He prepared vaccines. He examined and typed bacteria. He bred guinea pigs for his Wasserman reactions. He prepared histological specimens. He was responsible for the sterile syringe service.

An additional lab was provided for Dr Klein's biochemistry and histological work which was exciting in the days when Alzheimer's, Pick's and Jacob-Creutzfeld's diseases were pre-senile conditions and senile dementia was Senile Dementia. Before he became an administrator, Hemphill had taken considerable interest in Histology and Biochemistry and he was supportive of the maximum involvement of the lab in routine clinical work. The Path Lab was an important port of call in the medical pot boy's life.

Apart from the medical approach there were continuing attempts to improve patient social conditions. Visiting took place in the dining hall with a confusion of visitors limited to 2 per patient – a primitive undignified experience which entailed a multitude queuing outside the locked hospital gate on Wednesday and Sunday afternoon. This was changed to the previously unthinkable on-the-ward visiting. Relatives were not discouraged from expressing their justified dissatisfaction with ward conditions to officials of the Committee and to politicians or to anyone else who would listen. A feeling of therapeutic impotence although strong was countered by hope of impending change.

Ground "parole" was rapidly extended to large numbers of male patients who were then free to use the hospital estate for recreation. As the wards rapidly filled up with parole patients, the doors were unlocked. The use of parole became irrelevant.

Washing and bathing facilities began to be improved, outside lavatories were provided in the ward gardens and blast walls were being removed from the ward windows.

In 1944, the Board of Control noted the continuing success of a group of 30 of the most difficult and "refractory" male patients who were nursed together in the small ward (No 7), given as much individual attention as possible and all available privileges. "Outbreaks of violence have been almost eliminated. After a few months many patients hitherto intractable have been passed on to other wards to mix with the really well behaved patients." Next year in 1945 the Commissioners averred that "credit must be given to the male nurse in charge of the ward", the only Commissioners' entry which I have seen which praises an individual nurse. Actually they should have praised the two Charge Nurses of Ward 7, Tom (Bonzo)

Jones RMPA and Bill Jones RMPA (unrelated) who put their heads on the chopper more than half a century ago and whose praise was well deserved.

The problem of pulmonary tuberculosis was the clinical problem which was ever-present and which recurred most frequently and most urgently. The fear of "consumption" at the time was no less than the fear of cancer or of mental illness. Each year the statistics confirmed the persistent deadliness of phthisis. The disease was endemic in the hospital and was responsible for almost 10% of all hospital deaths. Hospital overcrowding and war time conditions rendered staff and patients increasingly vulnerable. Two male nurses and the medical superintendent had gone down with it in 1943.

There was no X-Ray department in the hospital. This limited the facilities for investigation. Dr Hemphill had returned to work whilst under the continuing care of Dr A. J. P. Alexander of Winsley Sanatorium near Bath, a physician of authority and compassion who undertook to advise on and to help with the Mental Hospital's problem. At this time mass miniature radiography (M.M.R.) had been introduced in Bristol. Dr E. E. Mawson, the Director of the M.M.R. unit, agreed to examine our patient population radiologically. For the first survey an immense amount of work was required to convey 1200 patients under war-time conditions 7 miles by bus to the (then) fixed M.M.R. unit at the Central Health Clinic. Future surveys were considerably less cumbersome in that the M.M.R. equipment was mobile and visited the hospital.

TABLE I.—*Results of Chest X-Ray Survey of Patients in Bristol Mental Hospital.*

	Males.		Females.		Total.	
	No.	%.	No.	%.	No.	%.
Total number in hospital during survey	540	—	700	—	1,240	—
„ „ sent for miniature radiography	512	94·8	669	95·6	1,181	95·2
„ „ who had large film three months before miniature film	20	3·7	7	1·0	27	2·2
„ „ who had large film subsequently	8	1·4	—	—	8	0·65
„ „ examined radiologically	540	100·0	676	96·6	1,216	98·1
„ „ not examined radiologically	—	—	24	3·4	24	1·9
„ „ with evidence of tubercle all stages	46	8·5	27	3·9	73	5·9
Active	13	2·4	4	0·6	17	1·4
1. Minimal lesions	1	0·2	—	—	1	0·08
2. Moderately advanced lesions	2	0·4	—	—	2	0·16
3. Far advanced lesions	10	1·9	4	0·6	14	1·1
Inactive	33	6·1	23	3·3	56	4·5
1. Minimal lesions	24	4·4	17	2·4	41	3·3
2. Moderately advanced lesions	9	1·7	6	0·9	15	1·2
3. Far advanced lesions	—	—	—	—	—	—
Doubtful lesions subsequently shown non-tuberculous	10	1·9	8	1·2	18	1·5
Pleural effusion	3	0·6	—	—	3	0·24
Non-tubercular lesions	21	3·9	25	3·6	46	3·7
Entirely negative	460	85·2	616	88·0	1,076	86·9

TABLE V.—*Radiographic Survey,* 1948.

1948.	Males.		Females.		Total.	
	Number.	%.	Number.	%.	Number.	%.
Patients in hospital	597	—	818	—	1415	—
„ X-rayed	592	99·2	791	96·7	1383	97·7
„ not X-rayed	5	0·8	27	3·3	32	2·3
Active tubercle	26	4·4	14	1·7	40	2·8
1. Minimal	9	1·5	6	0·7	15	1·1
2. Moderately advanced	8	1·3	5	0·6	13	0·9
3. Far advanced	9	1·5	3	0·4	12	0·8
Inactive tubercle (under observation)	24	4·0	11	1·3	35	2·5
Pleural involvement	1	0·2	—	—	1	0·1

Figure 42 The results of TB surveys in the Hospital

The results of the initial M.M.R. investigations and of the yearly surveys during the following 5 years were published in the Journal of Mental Science January 1946 and January 1950: In the initial 1944 survey there were 1240 patients in residence in the Bristol Mental Hospital. Sixty (60) patients, 30 in each of two buses were conveyed to each session assigned to us. In all 1181 patients attended. Those who had had X-rays within 3 months previously were not repeated (26 men, 7 women). Five hundred and twelve (512) men were examined, 100% of male patients and 669 women 96% of the females. The remainder being bed-ridden or very enfeebled or recently examined radiologically showed no clinical signs of tuberculosis. Eighty four (84) patients were recalled (51 male, 33 female) for large film examination and they were joined by 172 (77 male, 95 female) whose film was reported as doubtful for one reason or another. All of these had full clinical and laboratory investigation. Active disease was demonstrated in 13 men and in 4 women. In 1944 there was 100% uptake amongst staff 62 male nurses and administrative staff plus 58 female nurses, and 21 laundry, domestic and administrative staff. There was no significant disease discovered in the administrative or laundry staff. Three male nurses were subjected to further examination, 1 with a minimal new lesion was admitted to a sanatorium. Incidence amongst the nursing staff continued to be a nightmare. No active phthisis was shown amongst the female nurses in 1944 but one probationer nurse, negative at the time of the survey died of miliary tuberculosis within the following year. In 1945 a physician fell victim, a male nurse in 1946 and a male and female nurse in 1947.

Nurses working in sanatoria were well trained and safeguarded, but not those in general and mental hospitals. Fishponds nursing staff in contact with infected patients were seconded for a period of training to Winsley Sanatorium.

A new modern Phillips X-ray machine was ordered for the hospital, but owing to the delay in supply did not appear until Spring 1947. Subsequently in the active cases progress was checked radiologically every 3 months, and frequent clinical examinations were made.

Immediate provision of accommodation was urgent. An open veranda attached to the male infirmary ward was fitted with protective boarding against the weather providing separate "open air" accommodation of a crude, cold and uncomfortable kind. Existing veranda accommodation attached to the female infirmary ward was better than the male accommodation and served as a female sanatorium. Treatment was as far as possible along orthodox Sanatorium lines. Laundry was subject to steam sterilisation. Distinctive crockery and cutlery was provided and treated appropriately.

The question of providing central hospital accommodation was considered. Sanatorium beds for the general population were scarce and it was unlikely in 1945 that even a simple scheme would be undertaken locally for mentally ill patients. We could not conceive that 99 small units adequately staffed and equipped for treatment of patients would be provided in the 99 mental hospitals in England and Wales. If tackled piece meal each could at best provide a moderate service. We were convinced that the only satisfactory way of dealing with patient treatment and with nurse protection would be by the provision of a specialised unit serving the needs of several mental hospitals, modern sanatorium of 150 beds 2:1 male to female ratio. This could take into consideration the especial needs of psychiatric patients whose clinical care would be supervised by a Visiting Chest Physician with knowledge of the special problems of mental hospital practice and supported by psychiatrically qualified personnel trained in sanatorium routine. We proposed that the sanatoria be built in the field to the east of the 'Bristol Union Workhouse' just to the east of Fishponds Asylum. With the establishment of the N.H.S. in 1948 the development of a Regional Unit became a possibility. We laid a plan before the Regional Hospital Board. This was applauded but was overtaken by the development of specific treatment and tuberculosis became a less dangerous condition.

The incidence of active pulmonary tuberculosis remained high over the quinquenium 1944 – 1949 but there were no new cases amongst the hospital residents. The death rate expressed as a percentage of all hospital deaths reached one half of the pre-war rate. In 1948 only 2 patients died of pulmonary tuberculosis the lowest number ever recorded in hospital up to that time.

The conditions described prevailed in the pre-antibiotic era. Poverty, homelessness and drug resistance have brought phthisis once again to centre stage, with the fear that victims of poorly or unsupported community care will most likely be prominent victims of the modern menace of the old enemy and that long term psychiatric invalids may again be likely victims of this remorseless disease.

NOTES ON PROPOSED SANATORIUM

I) INTRODUCTION.

There is no doubt that such a sanatorium is urgently necessary. It is essential that it should be designed to allow Pulmonary Tuberculosis in mental hospitals to be treated along the most modern, enlightened and orthodox of sanatorium lines. If the building and equipment are not to be of the best, I consider that it would be better to make arrangements in such a hospital locally to deal with the problem.

I have worked throughout in the closest collaboration with Dr. A.J..P.Alexander of Winsley Sanatorium, and I enclose a personal letter which gives his views on the project.

II) GUIDING PRINCIPLES.

1) Location:

It will be seen by reference to the plans that the site of the proposed Tuberculosis sanatorium is situated within the hospital estate. See Ordnance Survey plan Glos. LXX 116, map reference 413.

2) The Nursing Problems:

This has been discussed with the officers concerned, the Matron and the Head Male Nurse. It is essential to have a building which can be nursed with the staff at present available. These officers assure me that the proposed buildings can be staffed adequately without any addition to their staff complements. (Dr Alexandra is willing to make arrangements for the training of staff.

3) The number of beds:

I discussed this question with Dr.Parr, Assistant Administrative Medical Officer to the Region. On the day of our conversation the official returns for Tuberculosis in mental hospitals in the northern half of the region were; 57 males and 7 females. These figures were obviously incorrect since on the same day we had returned 11 female patients.

The total number of mental hospital beds in the northern half of the region is approximately 6,300. If Stapleton Hospital be added the total becomes approximately 7,250. The number of cases of active Tuberculosis at Fishponds at present is 33(22 males and 11 females). Based on those figures 140 beds would be necessary in this sanatorium, or if Stapleton Hospital be added, 161 beds. The ratio of 2 males to 1 female is probably about correct. We have accordingly planned a unit of 149 beds, preserving this 2 –1 ratio.

Bristol Mental Hospitals	-	1,480
Gloucester Mental Hospitals	-	1,500
Wells Mental Hospital	-	1,000
Tone Vale Mental Hospital	-	900
Devizes Mental Hospital	-	1,450
Stapleton Hospital	-	900
Total	-	7,230

4) **Necessary Buildings**:
    1 Hospital Unit, Male.
    1 Hospital Unit, Female.
    1 Boiler House and O.T.D Unit.

III) GENERAL DESCRIPTION OF PROPOSED SANATORIUM.

1) We have planned separate blocks for male and female patients, with a separate Occupational Therapy Department adjoining both blocks.

2) Buildings:
a) Shape.
The Stellate design for the main buildings is proposed, after much consideration. The main points in favour of this design are that the area of land available is strictly limited; that nursing and observation with a restricted staff is more practicable; that adequate segregation of patients according to their mental categories is possible without separating them by long distances; that the medical and nursing treatment and administrative block is centrally situated and easy of access to all wards; and that the maximum number of wards have a southerly aspect.
b) Construction.
The wings of the male and female hospitals, together with the boiler house and occupation department, will be constructed of Orlit precast concrete, with verandas of precast concrete and glass. In-filling between the main structures will consist of concrete orlit blocks. The veranda side of the wings will consist mainly of the french window metal casement frames, as illustrated on page 14 of the orlit booklet.
The central sections of the male and female blocks will be carried out in standard building construction materials, outer walls facings of concrete blocks, and partition walls the usual brick construction.
The roof and whole building will be in reinforced concrete with provision for lighting and ventilation over the inner portion by means of lantern lights. The floors throughout the buildings will consist of mastic jointless flooring material with coved skirtings and walls will be in hard plaster finish with high gloss paint.
To prevent dust accumulation there will, as far as possible, be no pipe work or other projections on floors, walls, or ceilings.
Doors will be of the flush pattern

3) Engineering Services:

Heating:	The steam boiler, preferably of the electro type, will be situated together with the necessary pumps in the boiler house. This will supply steam to the laundry, kitchens, sterilising equipment and formelin room; also to the caloriferies. The heating system will consist of slow combustion acctional heating boiler, together with the necessary pumps, and the wards will be heated by the Ray Rad system, which will be incorporated in the ceilings.
Domestic Hot Water Supply:	Either by the electro method of thermal storage, or by a steam heated calorifier, together with the necessary storage containers.
Plumbing & Drainage	The plumbing and drainage will be carried out in the usual system, using standard equipment for mental hospitals. Drainage will be connected to the main sewer, which is running diagonally across the proposed site.
Electricity:	Ample lighting points and power points have been provided for, and special fittings for wards and dayrooms of the flush fitting type, with individual lighting for each bed.

IV) ROAD WORKS AND SERVICES.

A provisional sum has been allowed for the construction of roads and paths together with the lay-out of the grounds, as shown on the site plan.

V) SPECIAL FEATURES:

1) Areas and Cubic Space: Day and Night.
   The floor area of both the male and female dayrooms have been designed in excess of the Board of Control recommendations for the ordinary mental patient. This also gives a corresponding increase in cubic capacity.

   The same applies to the night dormitories, the same in this case being designed in excess of the recommendations of the Joint Tuberculosis Council.

2) Medical Services:
   Adequate clinical rooms are provided for. Which will be stocked with modern equipment. The X-ray department in the central building will be available.

3) Feeding Arrangements:
   It is proposed that patients should be fed from the central kitchen, the food being delivered from a separate door in the distributing kitchen, in heated conveyances. The Sanatorium kitchens are equipped to deal only with sick nursing diets.

4) The Shape of the Building
   The advantages are already described.

5) Verandahs:
   As far as possible with this type of construction we have made provision for verandahs of all blocks to face south. Ample space is allowed for accommodation of all bed patients on verandahs.

6) Single Rooms:
   These have been designed so as to afford observation from the dormitory and also from the corridor.

7) Day and Dining Rooms provided for each category:
   Day Rooms have been provided so that there is one for the "good" convalescent patients and another for the "bad" convalescent patients.
   The dining rooms have so been arranged that the "good" convalescent patients' dining room is situated to one side of the kitchen and the "bad" convalescent patients' dining rooms on the other side, thereby segregating the 2 categories of patients.

8) General Lay-out of Administrative Block:
   The administrative block is situated in the central part of the building and consists of the following rooms:
   Male Side: Medical Officer's Room; Visitor's Room; Clinic; Charge Nurse's Room; "Bad" Convalescent Patients' Dinning Room; "Bad" Convalescent Patients' Day Room; a Nurses' room, and a section set aside for staff cloak and dressing rooms.
   A Store is situated in the centre of the block, together with the necessary lavatory accommodation.
   The Female Side is the same as the Male Side, except that on the female side there is no day room in the central block.

   The Medical Officers' Room is situated near the Entrance Hall, with the clinic and visitors' room adjacent.
   The Visitors' Room has been designed so as to afford comfortable accommodation for visitors, having regard to the distance they may have to travel.

   Adequate provision has been made with regard to staff dressing room accommodation, and dressing rooms have been provided so that on coming staff change their clothing, and the clothing which they take off does not come into contact with that which they put on. Suitable built-in cupboards and drying facilities have been provided in these dressing rooms.

9) <u>Sanitary Annexes to Wards:</u>
Sanitary annexes have been provided between bed wards.

10) <u>Bathrooms:</u>
Provision has been made for a proportion of single bathrooms, together with a general bathroom with plastic curtaining between baths.

11) <u>Dressing Rooms and Adequate Wardrobe Space:</u>
Provision has been made for a dressing room to each Ward together with adequate wardrobe space.

12) <u>Storage:</u>
Provision has been made adequate storage space at the most convenient sections of the building.

13) <u>Occupational Therapy Department Block:</u>
After careful consideration with the Nursing Officers, a mixed occupational therapy block has been provided for. This block has a southerly aspect and is provided with a verandah. It is situated away from the main buildings and adjacent to the boiler house. Suitable lavatory accommodation, together with storage facilities has been allowed for.

14) <u>Airing Courts:</u>
Provision has been made for Airing Courts for the bad type of patient. These have been arranged on the extreme wings of the male and female blocks, so that only good patients on either side face one another.

15) <u>Laundry:</u>
Provision for a small foul and general laundry has been allowed for, adjacent to the boiler house. This will provide for sterile rough dried laundry for finishing in the main hospital laundry.

VI) **APPROXIMATE ESTIMATE OF COST**:

<u>Buildings:</u>

	£.	s.	d.
Female Sanatorium	48,000.	0.	0.
Male Sanatorium	69,000.	0.	0.
Boiler House, O.T.D.Dept., etc	8,500.	0.	0.
Engineering Services	18,500.	0.	0.
Laundry	1,500.	0.	0.
Furnishings & sundry equipment	9,050.	0.	0.
Roads & lay- out of grounds	7,900.	0.	0.
	£162,450.	0.	0.

NB   These figures may be compared with the following :-
1) Cheddleton Hospital built in 1893, cost per bed £ 280.00
2) Barrow Hospital built in 1937-38, cost per bed approx. £400

Peace and post-war problems

On May 8th 1945, V.E Day, patients and staff assembled in the Cinema Hall to hear Churchill declare the end of the war in Europe. There was an atmosphere of almost unbearable anticipation. Everywhere there was joyful turmoil. Bells, the wartime heralds of invasion, had not been heard for 5 years. The Fishponds Tower clock had struck neither hour nor quarter since muted for the Great War in 1914. At 3pm Henry Adams, the Hospital engineer, climbed into the belfry and manually struck the victory chime. This was their final peal. They were sold in 1952 and the clock was replaced by an electric timepiece. There followed dancing and a celebratory bonfire in the grounds of the Nurses Home.
On the next day reality returned. And it showed. The patients – men in particular – were looking very shabby. Clothes and footwear were getting scarce

There was continuing overcrowding – the average patient population in 1945 was 1222 – but relief in social conditions was promised when Barrow Hospital returned to City control.

The medical bustle grew apace. the Insulin Department treated 36 patients during the year. Miss Diana Kinlock-Beck, Consultant Neurosurgeon performed leucotomy on 15 patients and the out-patient service 3 days weekly in the B.R.I. saw 513 new patients plus 71 follow ups from hospital discharge. An x-ray department was promised and a 6 channel Electro-encephalogram was ordered.

The medical staff situation was changing rapidly. Pierce O'Malley joined in 1944 and returned to Belfast in 1946 via the National Hospital for Nervous Diseases, Queen Square to establish the first general hospital psychiatric unit in Ulster in the Mater Hospital Belfast. Desmond Pond was appointed Assistant Medical Officer, John Hawkings Clinical Assistant, Max Reiss Chief Research Biochemist, K.C.P.(Ken) Smith and C.R.G. (Bob) Howard, Registrars under the Government training scheme. New appointments to the Research Department followed in rapid succession.

The University of Bristol established a Diploma in Psychological Medicine and started a course in Autumn 1946. Relations with the Teaching Hospital and with the University appeared to be growing closer.

Shortage of female nurses was a continuing problem so serious that Hemphill averred that it was difficult to see how the work of the hospital could continue efficiently unless the female staff increased by at least 50%. Work was kept going only because it became possible to engage male porters to relieve female nurses of many non-nursing duties. The male staff situation improved as the men returned from the forces. The Radcliffe Committee's terms and conditions of service for the nursing staff were accepted and implemented.

In spite of everything the patient's social life improved. Cricket thrived under the captaincy of Dr K. C. P. Smith, football began again. The cinema was popular. Dances and concerts were well supported. The canteen had not yet recovered from the wartime scarcities but within limits, provided a fair service for patients and relatives.

Occupational therapy had a fillip: a therapist and 2 assistants were appointed for the female side. They were never provided with discrete accommodation but an unused annexe was converted into a makeshift department whilst the dining hall was used for up to 100 patients' during the winter. The men did marginally better when a large wooden ex-army hut, which was bought for £550 to provide a building for a patient' canteen, was diverted to O.T. Occupational therapy was never a well developed service in the hospital, nor did the O.T. staff ever exceed 5, 3 female and 2 male therapists, ill housed and poorly equipped, unable to make much impression on the idleness which was the curse of the hospital.

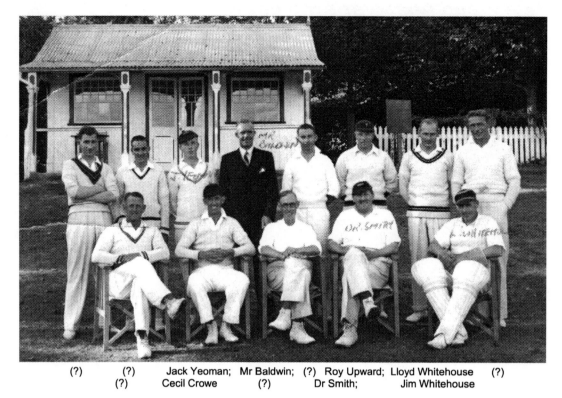

| (?) | (?) | Jack Yeoman; | Mr Baldwin; | (?) | Roy Upward; | Lloyd Whitehouse | (?) |
| | (?) | Cecil Crowe | (?) | | Dr Smith; | Jim Whitehouse | |

Figure 44   Glenside Cricket team at Tone Vale Hospital Sept 1967 - South Western Health Service Cup

The social work department was doubled by the appointment of Mrs Madge Grant. Jeanette Attlee was the first psychologist to join the staff. The sewing room was converted into an X-ray Department including a dark room and small waiting area. A former maids' dining room was fitted out as a photographic room.

Those connected with Management - the Visiting Committee, the Admin Staff, and the Board of Control - returned always to the problem of overcrowding which was daily more obvious. On 10th January 1946 the Commissioners ascribed the problem to the fact that "the Barrow Gurney division has not yet been handed back by the Naval Authorities." The Chairman of the Visiting Committee, Mr W. Dancy wrote in July of the same year that "the overcrowding of the wards continues to be a handicap to the efficiency of the hospital." He expressed the hope that when Barrow Hospital was released in Autumn 1946 "an early start will be made with the programme of ward reconstruction at Fishponds Hospital."

By mid 1946, the National Health Service Bill was before parliament. It occupied much of the staff conversation, discussion and argument. The problems of running a hospital as a group, Barrow / Fishponds, were well known from the difficulties experienced pre-war when Barrow ran in uneasy tandem with Fishponds for 16 months from May 1938 to September 1939. Hemphill often spoke of the then problems and was adamant that the mistakes of the past should not be repeated. Some of the staff especially those interested in the treatment of psychoses and of organic conditions, listened, with some doubt, to the repeated assurances of the Visiting Committee, the Commissioners and the Medical Superintendent but hope was bolstered by their repeated affirmations and by the declared intentions of the administrators, the researchers and the clinicians.

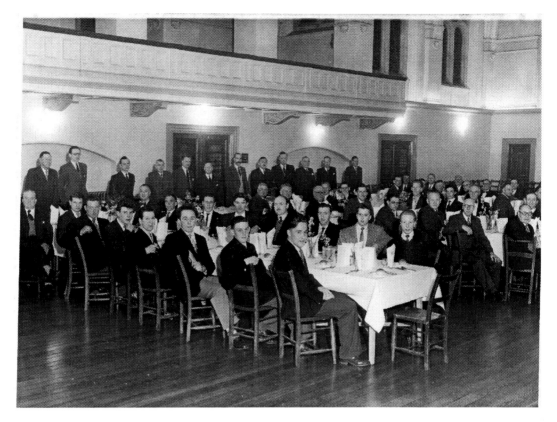

Figure 45 Second A.F.C. Dinner May 1957

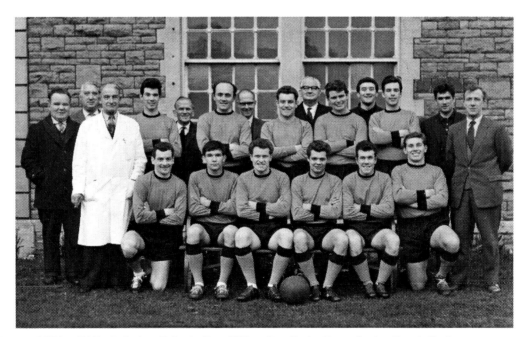

Dennis Griffiths; Sid Nash; Sydney Roberts; Dave Withey; Reg Davis; Roger Gunter; Francis Coates; →
→ Des Tight; Lewis Walker; Mike Rogers; Terry Martin; Alan Withey; Jeff Mansfield; Jimmy Adams
Dave Sherman; Bradly Mansfield; Bob Dace; Beverley Reynolds; Fred Dace; Alan Smith

The photograph includes three sets of brothers.

Figure 46 Football Team for 1963-4 season Gloucester Senior Cup Final

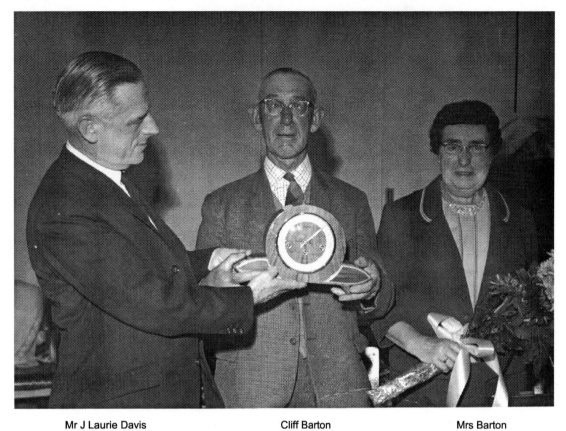

| Mr J Laurie Davis | Cliff Barton | Mrs Barton |

Figure 47 Presentation at Cliff Barton's Retirement 26th Sept. 1969

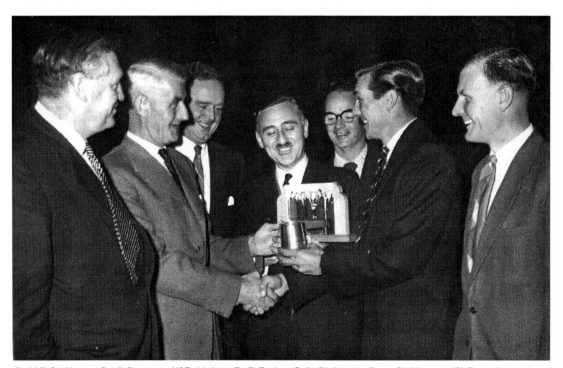

| Dr K P Smith | Cecil Crowe | Alf Baldwin | Dr D Early | Colin Binham | Dave Smith | (?) Reporter |

Figure 48 Dinner Pre-M.C.C. Tour (Dave Smith) May 1957

Of future local plans for the N.H.S. Hemphill wrote in July 1946

> Bristol as a University City will be the key of the South West Region. As a centre of psychiatry it is well favoured, having a modern hospital at Barrow Gurney as well as the older mental hospital at Fishponds... Barrow Hospital could become a centre for research and training for which its method of construction make it suitable... In anticipation of the return of Barrow the research programme at Fishponds is being expanded, the technical staff are being engaged and essential equipment is being installed. It should be possible to have a comprehensive psychiatric service in Bristol with an outstanding research, teaching and treatment Institute. However, the older hospital at Fishponds is badly in need of modernisation and at first, part of Barrow will have to be used for the overflow from Fishponds. The construction of new Admission Blocks at Fishponds, an extension of the Nurses Home and the breaking up of the larger wards into smaller units, have been the subject of report and discussion by the Visiting Committee. They have approved the principle that the older hospital should not be allowed to deteriorate into an institute for chronic patients but should function as a mental hospital, although perhaps less specialised than Barrow.

No-one knew exactly what to expect when Barrow returned to civilian occupation. The hospital was the most modern mental hospital building in the country, greatly appreciated by the City of Bristol who appointed a new Committee of Visitors under a socialist Chairman and who gave indications that they regarded the hospital as a valuable and prestigious asset to be treated generously.

As early as 1939, Dr J. J. B. Martin the then Medical Superintendent asserted that Barrow was undoubtedly a great advance in that "the early case will have fair and adequate treatment" and that it would allow a temporary solution to the overcrowding at Fishponds. His main criticism was, the intersection of the hospital grounds by ditches, together with the dense woodland which were dangerous for mental patients The Ordnance Survey map referred to the Barrow site as " the Wild Country" to which access was gained via Wild Country Lane. He also commented on the poor social amenities which were provided for patients and staff.

There were, however, many other difficulties which Dr Hemphill had personally experienced in 1938/39. Most importantly the practical problems of interpersonal relationships between staff in isolated conditions. He had often spoken of the unpleasant disagreements pre-war between Fishponds and Barrow and he avowed that such bitterness should not be allowed to recur. The co-operative arrangements proposed in his report to the Visiting Committee in July 1946 were enthusiastically endorsed by old and new medical staff. Fishponds was to be an active clinical unit and was not to deteriorate into an oubliette. This was a determining factor in the high morale amongst all grades of staff whilst awaiting the re-opening of Barrow.

These were the functions proposed for Fishponds: the treatment of cases of schizophrenia, supported by the established Insulin Department would ensure a steady admission of young patients with acute mental illness. Admission for other diagnostic categories to be offered for their convenience to patients from the North side of the City if they so wished. Patients suffering from tuberculosis were to have a villa in Barrow laid aside for them until a special unit could be built in Fishponds, whilst the treatment of and research into the more chronic mental illnesses associated with long stay were to be developed in Fishponds.

Meanwhile, the Board of Control paid tribute to the spirit of progress in Fishponds whilst expressing disquiet about overcrowding. The hospital resources were strained to the limit, sanitary and toilet facilities were 'painfully inadequate'. Patients clothing continued to deteriorate. Clinical evaluation, physical and mental, was lauded by the Commissioners. The Insulin Department treated 59 patients in 1946, pre-frontal leucotomy was carried out on 32 patients. New machines for electro-convulsive treatments were introduced. Electronarcosis was found to be ineffective and potentially dangerous and was abandoned. Penicillin had arrived. Therapeutic malaria had had its day.

The Research Department, established in 1945, the jewel in the post-war crown was enthusiastically supported. In 1946 Hemphill wrote "In establishing a research department, the Visiting Committee have introduced a most outstanding development in the history of the hospital… It has been possible in less than a year to build up a really valuable unit for biochemical and physiological research into the causation of mental illness, of a quality and size scarcely equalled by any other mental hospital in the country." He rightly claimed that the project was welcomed by all the hospital staff.

In Barrow Hospital preparations for civilian occupation proceeded. Dr John Hawkings, vigorously undertook the medical re-equipment. There was little discussion about policy or strategy. The choice of professional, artisan and administrative staff for Barrow was carried out on an *ad hoc* basis. No one knew how decisions were being made nor how questions of staff location were decided. This led to some disgruntled restlessness. Two non-medical psychologists were appointed and resigned within a year. Dr Garmany, the Deputy Medical Superintendent and Assistant Lecturer in Psychiatry in the University of Bristol resigned and became Regional Psychiatrist to the South West Metropolitan Regional Hospital Board. He was replaced by Dr G. A. Fraser Steele who had been Acting Deputy Medical Director at Jordanbourn Nerve Hospital and Lecturer in Psychiatry, Edinburgh University. Dr K. C. P. Smith resigned to go into general practice. Desmond Pond, resigned on medical grounds. Five other doctors Thomas, Maggs, Stuart, Bickford and Crotty joined the staff in 1946/47, Dr Thomas was in charge of the newly-opened Department of Electro-encephalography, but he too emigrated ere long.

Others came and went. Some who stayed had considerable doubts about the way the wind was blowing. Ken Smith remarked that Bristol had turned out some good psychiatrists. He caricatured one of these who stayed behind which temporarily raised our spirits.

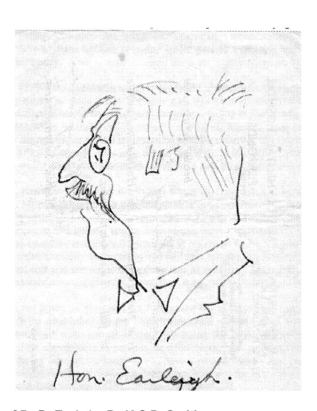

Figure 49 Sketch of Dr D. Early by Dr K.C.P. Smith

Research – Decline & Fall

The birth of the Research Department was not without difficulty. The Visiting Committee gave vigorous encouragement and support. By the time that Max Reiss was appointed Research Consultant relations between Fishponds and the Burden Neurological Institute were strained.

The medical staff had visionary thoughts of a fundamental break through and the nursing staff shared this optimism. In the late 1940's the Department imbued excitement and expectancy into the clinical work of the hospital.

In the early days the department in Fishponds grew rapidly with support from the Works Department, whose staff produced brilliant laboratory conditions and equipment from unpromising materials. Much of the credit for this was due to Mr H. A. Adams, Hospital Engineer and to his staff, who manufactured laboratory benches, apparatus and fittings mostly out of scrap and who planned the water, lighting, heating and steam services from severely restricted supplies. The facilities were remarkable. Five laboratories provided by converting an old kitchen, a maid's sitting room, a disused part of the laundry and a boiler house, were equipped for specialist work and an animal house was constructed for keeping and for breeding upwards of 2000 Wistar rats and a number of rabbits.

Steam laid on to several benches elicited the enthusiastic declaration by Max Reiss to a visiting guest "Everything here will steam!

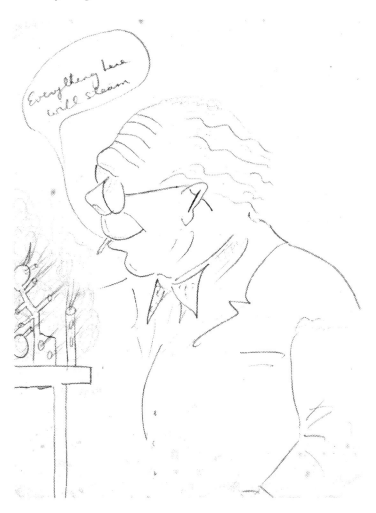

Figure 51 Biochemical laboratory by K C P Smith

The staff by the end of the first year numbered 15, one senior biochemist, Dr J. J. Gordon, three biochemists, five senior technicians and six junior technicians. The principal lines of investigation were into endocrine changes in schizophrenia and in manic depressive psychosis, vitamin content of various organs, measurement of protein bound iodine in blood as an indicator of thyroid activity and experimental investigation in rats of the mode of action of electro-convulsive activity.

By the end of 1947 no tangible results were being reported in spite of a large number of patients having undergone investigation. Hemphill reported that "it had been found that certain lines of research must be done on a larger scale." Plans were made for extensive laboratory development at Barrow although "there (was) at Fishponds the largest department for biochemical and endocrinological research in mental diseases in the country."

Bit by bit, the department was moved to Barrow. By the early 1950's, co-operation between clinicians and research workers was deteriorating. The laboratories were becoming increasingly divorced from their original purpose of clinical research. As the hopes of favourable results dwindled, cynicism was growing, particularly amongst the nursing staff. As late as 1951 Hemphill was still hoping that "a successful outcome of research in any one disease group in Psychiatry would alter the position enormously."

As time went on it became increasingly questionable whether the claims for correlation between psychiatric symptoms and laboratory findings were tenable. The Lab results of 24hour specimens of urine, for the measurement of total and fractional keto-steriods, appeared to nurses to have little to do with patients' clinical states, although research workers sometimes made extravagant clinical claims to the contrary. This sometimes led to poor co-operation between the clinicians and the research workers who then pursued lines of research divorced from their original purpose. In Fishponds, there were neither routine meetings nor conferences to discuss and to control projects nor was there much attempt to provide information to the research workers about patients' clinical conditions, their diagnosis, treatment and the course of their illness. Nursing staff who initially were keen and co-operative became sceptical, especially when their work in specimen collection, in supervision and control of patients was criticised.

The reputation of the department, although waning, was boosted in 1950, when the Society of Endocrinology held their annual meeting at Barrow Hospital. Organon Laboratories described the adrenocorticotrophic hormone (A.C.T.H.) manufactured in Reiss' laboratory as 10% to 15% more active biologically than their commercially produced product. Reiss, was awarded a D.Sc. by Bristol University for his work. His standing was high and the continuing production of A.C.T.H. maintained credibility in his department. His status depended on his recognition by the University, by Industry and by his immediate colleagues who appreciated his genius which amongst other things had enabled him to produce his A.C.T.H. in the Fishponds laboratory from pigs' pituitary glands collected weekly from Harris' Bacon Factory in Calne (Wiltshire). His methods of standardisation of this substance were accepted by the Medical Research Council and 25gms of his Z3 preparation were supplied to their Biological Standards and retained provisionally as the British Standard. The substance prepared in Bristol labs continued to be used for scientific purposes and for response testing until 1956.

In 1952 a 4 year survey of the work of the Research Department was written by the Medical Superintendent, not by Max Reiss, the Consultant in charge of the department. The report introduced itself by describing a fire in the Ketosteroid lab in December 1951, when a benzene container burst. This dramatic event introduced a re-statement of the direction being pursued by research – "to define endocrine and other patho-physiological components of mental illness, of mental functioning and of emotion; to direct treatment to the basis of patho-physiological analysis; to pursue research in the properties of hormones and steroids and to develop better and more precise methods of laboratory and clinical investigations."

The doubts of the clinicians could no longer be dismissed. An attempt was made to re-state the direction of the research and to make the best case possible for progress. The survey was often exaggerated and inaccurate The statement that radio-active thyroid investigation using the ring counter designed by Haigh had come into routine clinical use in the majority of admissions was not applicable to Fishponds, nor was the claim that the results often pointed the way to further analysis and to appropriate treatment, nor did results lead to enlightenment "in problems of thyroid function in anxiety as well as in other disorders." Adrenal function tests adapted and modified by the department were also claimed to have passed into clinical use and to be "providing information about the physiological mechanisms of shock therapies and of recurrent mental disorders." As far as Fishponds was concerned they hadn't and they didn't. Nor did anterior pituitary hormone prepared and standardised in the laboratory prove to be useful "in the treatment of patients on the basis of hormone analysis." Nor did measurements of the total and fractional keto-steroids become part of the clinical routine nor did the "other investigations mentioned allow a more complete picture of physiological interconnections in psychiatric illness to be obtained than has hitherto been possible."

The end of the 1952 report made doubtfully sustainable clinical claims, and many explanatory excuses which presaged disaster. Amongst them were complaints that the number of beds set aside for research in Barrow (12 male, 14 female) "are practically useless for statistical evaluation", a unit with so few beds being "totally unsatisfactory", and that "separation of labs in Barrow and Fishponds was inconvenient and made it inevitable that new buildings such as an animal house should be erected in Barrow." Clinical evaluation of patients was said to be made difficult by the degree of severity and the duration of the illness and by the great variation those patients suffering from apparently the same disorder, which called for great caution in deciding the correlation between lab findings and symptoms. There was criticism of nursing standards maintaining that "there were many disappointments due to incomplete urine collections and to lack of proper supervision and control of conditions in which patients are nursed."

With hindsight the excuses appear to be a preparation for admission of failure. A long paragraph presented a retrospect of 4 years work, which maintained that "some real progress appears to have been made in defining the physiology of mental states and in adapting modern methods of their elucidation. No dramatic results... By comparison with Insulin and ECT the effective dosage of hormones so far used is very small ... It may be that to avoid some of the disagreeable results of shock treatments, hormone therapy, less violent, may have to be continued over a much longer period than is at present usual."

Therapeutic trials, it was claimed, were handicapped by the difficulty in establishing criteria for improvement, as well as by the severity of the illness; "every refinement in laboratory measurements should be accompanied by refinements in assessment of the meaning of human behaviour and of dynamics in the psychological sphere." The report later points out the difficulty applying the results of animal work to humans so that "the research institute that relies on animals will contribute much academic phenomenology but may even mislead when the results are translated into terms of clinical practise with humans."

As the report progresses to 5½ pages it becomes more discursive. It avers that research is very expensive but claims that even more money could be wisely spent in developing and devising methods of physiological evaluation of the mentally sick. The view is expressed that studies in psychosomatic medicine are desirable but are impossible without altering the environment of the experiments although investigations need not be unduly extravagant.

The hopes of the Department were finally shattered in 1955 as described in the decennial hospital report by the Medical Superintendent in 1959, which dismissed the great Biochemical and Endocrine Research Department in 2 paragraphs:

> Research in physiology, biochemistry and endocrinology of mental disorders was initiated during the war and in 1946 Dr Max Reiss was appointed to direct the laboratory work. During the next 10 years some research laboratories were constructed and other buildings converted as such at Fishponds and Barrow hospitals.

A large amount of work was carried out, particularly in schizophrenia and some promising lines were pursued. As the work became more complex the department expanded until over 30 workers were employed. A large proportion of the effort was then being devoted to pharmacological problems, such as the properties, method of production and standardisation of hormones. These highly specialised subjects require well-qualified senior research workers, of whom there was a great shortage. The Regional Board had to give consideration to these questions and in 1955 the Research Department was taken from the Bristol Mental Hospital and renamed "The Biochemical and Endocrinological Research Unit of the South Western Regional Hospital Board." As the Medical Research Council apparently was not prepared to take over the unit, it was closed down in March 1957, the staff was disbanded, the laboratories converted to other uses and the apparatus dispersed to various hospitals. This was a matter of great regret, for much valuable preparatory work was lost and facilities for biochemical research came to an end. The medical staff was unsuccessful in having any part in this research department preserved. Research on similar lines is yielding promising results in other psychiatric institutes.

The demise of the department was slow and excruciatingly painful. Old friendships were shattered and the final disbursement of laboratory equipment was unsavoury in the wolfish rapacity of the predators who gorged themselves on the misfortune of their colleagues. A sense of relief ultimately accompanied the final melancholy curtain.

The Re-Opening of Barrow Hospital 1947

Staffing difficulties

The Royal Navy handed Barrow back to Bristol Corporation in January 1947.

In July, when already partially occupied by patients, Mr M W Dancy, Chairman of the Visiting Committee expressed the hope that "the plans already made for both hospitals will be brought to fruition by our successors." Under N.H.S. management (1948) he was to be replaced by Alderman Burgess as Chairman of the newly established Hospital Management Committee.

Other major staff changes were taking place. Mr Herbert A. Wilkins who had been Clerk and Steward since 1906 was replaced in 1947 by Mr J. L. (Laurie) Davis who thus became the last Clerk and Steward (From Issue No.90 of *The Glensider*, on 12th August 1971: "Do you remember?" Our former Clerk and Steward (Secretary) Mr Herbert Wilkins whose period of service extended from April 1906 to April 1947? Congratulations on 80th birthday – 8th August 1971) to the Visiting Committee and on the Appointed Day 4th July 1948 the first Secretary of the Hospital Management Committee. Mr Chambers who had been Mr Wilkins' deputy retired at the same time after 32 years service.

Hemphill wrote that the opening of Barrow in July 1947 had been just possible without depleting Fishponds staff to the point of danger. He wrote that "departments for psychological investigation, electro-encephalography and physiological research will be set up, (in Barrow) so that in the first week after admission, accurate diagnosis and a correct line of treatment can be established." He added that research would continue "in the present way" in Fishponds "the largest department of endocrine and biochemical research in mental disorders in the country" and that a close liaison between the two hospitals would continue.

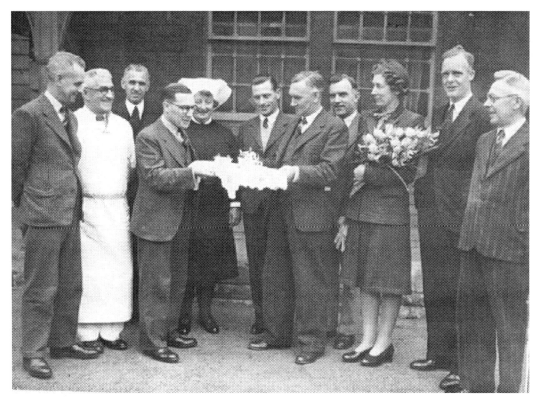

Figure 52 The End of an Era - Mr H A Wilkins retires 1947

Before Barrow re-opened, policy agreements were agreed informally, no hard and fast rules had been written down. Very soon, undiscussed decisions by the Medical Superintendent began to make clinical management of Fishponds very difficult. It was not until 22nd March 1948 that a written admission policy was reluctantly provided. It ordered that all patients would be admitted to Barrow except known mental defectives, chronic psychotics, chronic epileptics, seniles and infectious cases (including TB).

22nd March, 1948.

<u>*ADMISSIONS*</u>
For the time being all patients, both Certified and Voluntary, will be admitted to Barrow Hospital except the following categories:-

1.   Known mental defectives.
2.   Known chronic psychotics.
3.   Known chronic epileptics.
4.   Seniles.
5.   Infective cases (including T.B.)

These categories will be admitted direct to Fishponds.

A Medical Officer will visit Stapleton Institution on Monday and Thursdays, or whenever certification of a patient is contemplated in order to decide where the patient is to be admitted.

It is desirable for patients to arrive at Barrow Hospital on Mondays and Thursdays at about 11 a.m. if possible.

Medical Superintendent.

In Barrow an instruction was issued in July 1948 that "Barrow should act as an admission centre for the investigation of all new cases and for the treatment of recoverable cases." These instructions ran counter to the expressed intentions and assurances of the Visiting Committee, which determined in 1945 that "the older hospital must not be allowed to deteriorate into an institute for chronic patients but should function as a modern hospital." They spelled the end of Fishponds as an active hospital. Neither medical nor senior nursing nor administrative staff were in a position to raise any objection to this directive and neither the Regional Hospital Board (of which Dr Hemphill was a member) nor the newly appointed Hospital Management Committee chose to suggest any different arrangement. The Group, therefore, was not to function by agreement and it seemed likely that the large hospital would become a dependent satellite of the smaller Barrow, with little influence on its own management or future development.

An atmosphere of distrust began to pervade relationships as the staffing of Barrow was taking shape. There was to be a fair allocation of staff of all disciplines. In fact, from the start the medical professional staffing situation developed to the detriment of Fishponds. Nominally fair shares applied also to nurses. Fishponds relied on the Matron and the Chief Male Nurse to employ and to allocate sufficient nursing and ancillary staff to maintain a good standard of patient care. The nursing administration tried to be fair but no staff/patient ratio was ever agreed and the female nursing staff level was dangerously low, so that ward care was always in a precarious state. The female nursing staff turnover in 1946 was more than 100%. Male staffing was generally more stable and was reasonably good.

Ward maintenance in Fishponds was neglected "None of the overdue and very necessary alterations in the wards of Fishponds was carried out" whereas in Barrow "complete redecoration both inside and out" followed de-requisition by the Admiralty.

Departments whose services were previously provided in other locations were called in to Barrow, such as the Out-patient E.C.T. Clinic at 12 Grove Road and the Social Workers Department. The proposed arrangement to provide humane facilities for the in-patient treatment of pulmonary tuberculosis in Barrow was withdrawn. The agreement to continue the Insulin Department in Fishponds was revoked and the department was transferred to Barrow. The new Department of experimental and Applied Psychology made no provision for services to Fishponds nor did the Department of Electroencephalography.

The main strength of the re-opened Barrow was that it was a modern hospital. However, it was inconveniently situated on the south side of the city 11 miles from Fishponds Hospital and had poor social amenities. Only a quarter of the original hospital building plan had been completed and thus there was an imbalance between the types of accommodation provided, e.g. there was a 100 bedded infirmary unit, which had been designed for the needs of an old fashioned mental hospital of 1,200 patients. Furthermore, the electrical supply was D.C., which gave rise to great problems with equipment, domestic and scientific, particularly apparatus such as E.C.T. and E.E.G.

The administrative staff – the Secretary, Laurie Davis, and the deputy Secretary Norman Kearns had headquarters in Glenside with another deputy Hospital Secretary in Barrow. Laurie Davis gathered around him a good, effective team and ran a concerned patient-orientated administration. Henry Adams, the Hospital engineer had his HQ in Glenside and he was responsible for the management of the hospital artisan and engineering staff. He found it difficult to balance the Fishponds/Barrow equation but continually strove to improve living conditions in Fishponds and consistently opposed the 'lick and promise' approach.

The year leading up to the N.H.S. was a trying one nationally for hospital staff. Medical staff was particularly vulnerable, Fishponds was no exception. Professional grading to decide personal N.H.S. status was an unnerving experience for each doctor except those in charge of departments. The process gave rise to mistrust of the Ministry's innominate advisors and to grave anxiety for a majority of medical staff. In Adult Psychiatry, only the Medical Superintendent of the Mental Hospital was graded as a Consultant. I was appointed physician in charge of Fishponds Hospital in 1947 and was responsible for the clinical administration of 1200 plus beds. I was graded as a Senior Registrar which being a training grade was clearly inappropriate. I refused an offer of re-grading to Senior Hospital Medical Officer (S.H.M.O.) and retained conditions enjoyed whilst in the pre-NHS employment of the Corporation. From 1947 to 1951, I was responsible for the clinical management of the hospital whilst in a non-consultant job. This situation improved in 1951, when I was appointed to consultant status, and when later invited by the Chairman to attend the H.M.C. and its sub-committees in an advisory capacity. The first evident consequence of this was the H.M.C.'s agreement at my request to place a limit of 1185 on the spiralling number of beds in the hospital.

Dr Grant with 15 years hospital experience and the only other senior doctor in Fishponds was initially graded a Junior Hospital Medical Officer (J.H.M.O.), changed on appeal to Senior Hospital Medical Officer (S.H.M.O), a non-consultant permanent grade. In addition there was on the staff of Fishponds a Junior Hospital Medical Officer, a Senior House Officer and sometimes a trainee. The method of allocation of staff too was capricious and continued to give rise to dissatisfaction especially when a doctor transferred from Barrow to Fishponds interpreted the change as demotion or as a punishment. Dr Robert Klein was allocated to the staff of Barrow on its re-commissioning. He was given an office there and access to a laboratory where he carried on his neurological research work. Within the year he was requested to return to work in Fishponds. He was not aware of the reason for this move. Whilst he was away, difficult staff decisions had been made in Fishponds and he returned to find the routine re-organised within a very tight schedule. Before his move to Barrow he was willingly accorded a privileged investigative and clinical position which was no longer possible. He resigned and took up an appointment at Crichton Royal Hospital, Dumfries. Bristol thus lost a brilliant neurologist, a friend and a gentle man, together with his family. This event was most traumatic to him and to his friends. It was only one of many such episodes caused by apparently erratic decision making.

Barrow Hospital expanded rapidly. Supported by excellent medical staff and growing facilities it provided an increasingly good clinical service. Fishponds Hospital struggled to survive, whilst adhering to its imposed commitments. The disposal of medical staff was in the hands of the Medical Superintendent. From the re-opening of Barrow in 1947, Fishponds was left to get on with it medically, supported by senior assistant medical officer (M.O.), a junior M.O. and 1 or 2 trainees. With formal grading in July 1948 – the Appointed Day for the N.H.S. – these titles changed to Senior Hospital Medical Officer (S.H.M.O.), Junior Hospital Medical Officer (J.H.M.O.) and 1 or 2 Senior House Officers (trainees). In other departments, nursing, maintenance, finance and admin, there was never a sufficient budget and at times they were compelled to leave work undone in Fishponds, so as to proceed in Barrow.

Morale was difficult to maintain. It was hard to assure the remaining staff that anything other than second-class status was in store for the Fishponds patients and staff. K. C. P. Smith portrayed a bleaker climate, interpreted a different mood.

The level of medical staffing continued to give rise to dissent for years to come. If the long continuing saga be told at this juncture, the continuing story of the hospital will then flow more evenly without the constant recurrence of references to this unpalatable subject.

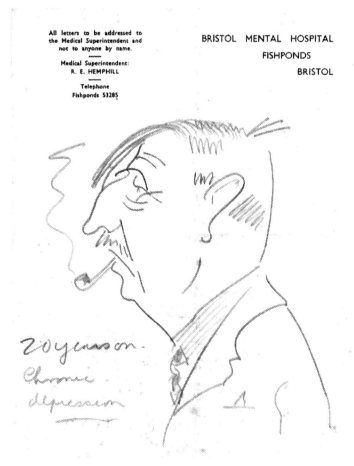

Figure 53 Dr K C P Smith caricatured a bleaker climate in 1948

In 1951 there were 20 doctors on the Fishponds/Barrow staff. In Barrow there were 5 Consultants, three S.H.M.O.'s, one J.H.M.O., two Senior Registrars and four Registrars – 15 in all. In Fishponds – 1 Consultant, one S.H.M.O.(Dr Grant) one J.H.M.O. and two S.H.O. This was the pattern which was firmly established but never agreed to after the establishment of the N.H.S..

In 1955, a second Consultant was appointed on the Fishponds Staff. Dr. Robert Martlew of Rainhill Hospital, Liverpool brought a new dimension to the life of the hospital. He contributed knowledge, wisdom, humanity and humour to patients and colleagues alike. He achieved many advances during his brief stay. After 18 months he returned to Liverpool as Deputy Superintendent at Rainhill to his friend Dr Finkleman, whom he later succeeded as Medical Superintendent.

Medical staff discrimination continued. In 1958, medical salaries in Fishponds cost 3/- [15p] per patient per week; in Barrow £1:0:6d. [£1.03]. Neville Lancaster, one of the Barrow consultants offered 2 sessions per week to help Fishponds. His offer was conditional on other changes and was not accepted by the Board. Dr Kelly the Senior Administrative Medical Officer of the Board, asked for information about integration of Fishponds/Barrow medical staff. There was none to give

On 21st July 1958, out of the blue the Secretary of the Regional Hospital Board wrote to J. L. Davis the hospital secretary to inform him that the Board had decided in principle that the existing staffing of the hospital was to be altered and that each hospital was to have its own medical superintendent. On the following day, the H.M.C. having asked all of its officers except the Hospital Secretary to withdraw from their meeting considered this unheralded bombshell and asked for more information and for an interview with the R.H.B..

On 25th July, Dr Kelly wrote to Dr Hemphill explaining that the Board intended to reorganise the hospitals so that Fishponds and Barrow each had its own medical superintendent. Many letters, meetings, and memos, statements form a vast archive concerning the ensuing controversies. It is difficult to summarise them or to describe the atmosphere which bedevilled the hospital for the years to come.

The H.M.C. met members of the Regional Hospital Board in private and then formally convened on 28th October 1958 in private session without officers except the Hospital Secretary. I asked them to hear the Fishponds view on the medical staff allocation before reaching a decision, which they did. This was the only occasion on which this point of view was expressed to the Committee. They were sympathetic; the Chairman was congratulatory on the presentation of Fishponds case. The Hospital Management Committee by a majority of 6 to 3 resolved "that this Committee concurs with the Boards proposal that the present arrangements be altered so that separate medical superintendents be appointed to Fishponds and Barrow Hospital." This motion was acknowledged by the R.H.B. and the Ministry of Health was informed.

At the next meeting of the H.M.C. on 25th November, I did not attend. There was a suggestion that the Medical Superintendent withdraw and a counter motion that he should stay. He remained. Two members proposed and another supported the motion for recession of the motion of 28th October, which its supporters said "would be tantamount to a vote of no confidence in the medical superintendent." It was decided that further discussion was necessary. The H.M.C. constituted itself a subcommittee and arranged to meet on 9th December. They considered the Board's memorandum paragraph by paragraph with comments by the medical superintendent. The motion of 28th October of concurrence with the Board's proposals was again proposed and passed by 8 votes to 3. This decision was relayed to the Board on January 7th 1959.

On 9th February 1959 the R. H. Board informed the hospital secretary that the Minister of Health had no objection and requested without delay a statement of administrative changes.

On 9th March each senior Hospital Departmental Head indicated no objection to medical separation; no problem was foreseen in any department.

The R.H.B. was so informed. But then they started to dither. The Mental Health Committee of the Board had become interested and the Senior Administrative Medical Officer asked for information on behalf of its Chairman. By mid July, the R.H.B. Secretary wrote that it was "the intention of the Board that both hospitals should accept patients of all age groups and clinical categories" and suggested that "one method of achieving this would be to agree catchment areas for each hospital", a suggestion which found favour with none at the time.

By the end of November the original plan for medical separation gave way to an offer of 2 sessions per week at Fishponds by Barrow consultants Dr Leitch and Dr Valentine, each in charge of 350 long stay beds "assisted by a Senior Hospital Medical Officer, a senior registrar about half-time with a registrar and junior working full-time." The Board had apparently lost enthusiasm for radical change and by April 1960 Dr Kelly talked of implementing the interchange of medical staff between Barrow and Fishponds "as agreed during our discussions of 21st March." There was in fact no such agreement.

The Board had had enough of the Bristol Mental Hospitals and when Professor Coutts, Chairman of the Mental Health Committee of the R.H.B., a Law Professor at Bristol University, Professor Neale, Professor of Paediatrics at Bristol University and Mr J. R. Mackie, a retired Colonial Administrator were asked to review staffing of all the regional psychiatric hospitals, the Establishment Committee asked that the Barrow/Glenside problem be referred to them. In February 1961 they produced their recommendations, amongst which were that if Dr Hemphill wished to continue to be designated as Medical Superintendent this should be limited to Barrow Hospital/Dundry Villa, and that a medical superintendent should not be appointed to Glenside Hospital nor to the Day Hospital. The H.M.C regarded the Mental Health Committee's suggestion as unworkable and again sought an internal solution.

A joint programme was proposed by the H.M.C. but the Board imposed its plan and Drs Leitch, Lancaster and Valentine started work in Glenside in July 1961.

And so for the first time in 13 years apart from Dr Martlew's 18 month stint, the old hospital (Fishponds) with its 1200 beds had more than one consultant psychiatrist working there. Dr Leitch was responsible for 300 beds, Dr Lancaster for 259 and Dr Valentine for 300, all mainly long stay or "chronic" patients. Sessional time allocated to all three of them added together amounted to a little over half of a full time consultant, Drs Lancaster and Leitch started Out-Patients at Southmead (General) Hospital and Dr Valentine at Frenchay (General) Hospital. In the first 2 years, 1962 and 1963 between them they were responsible for 30% of all admissions to Glenside. Dr Lancaster and Dr Leitch were not satisfied with their allotted bed complement and the medical staff situation was still so unbalanced that the Establishment Committee acknowledged the situation and in November 1964 decided to review again the working of the team system. This resulted in no significant change.

The establishment of a Chair of Mental health in the University of Bristol in 1965 led to the location of an undergraduate Teaching Unit in Glenside Hospital. Professor Derek Russell-Davis and his deputy Dr John Roberts admitted a small number of patients to the unit, which helped little to lighten the clinical load. It had the effect of incorporating Glenside in undergraduate and post-graduate training and for the first time a Senior Registrar was attached to the Fishponds Department of Social Psychiatry. The Board's medical staffing formula for Glenside continued as before.

On 11th March 1966, the Establishment Committee again constituted their sub-committee under the Chairmanship of Professor Neale, once more to consider the medical staffing of Glenside Hospital. The atmosphere of the meeting was cool but not acrimonious. No agreement was possible and the Board members became evidently irritated by the failure of the consultants to come to a compromise.

Professor Neale pressed for my opinion on the shortcomings of the established arrangements. I was reluctant to express any view which was likely to be taken as personal criticism of colleagues. Professor Neale persisted again and again. I then averred that patients got less doctor time than when the old regulations prevailed and when by law each patient was examined regularly twice yearly, thus ensuring that none got "lost" in the crowd. I also informed him that doctors in my team had spoken of frequently being required to attend to the needs of patients under the care of other teams in the absence of their own medical advisor.

These statements aroused a bitterness of feeling which was represented to Mr English (later Sir John), the Chairman of the Regional Hospital Board on 28th March 1966 in a document signed by the five consultants, led by the signature of Dr. R. E. Hemphill (Medical Superintendent). All of these doctors spent the greater part of their time working in Barrow Hospital, two of them did not work at all in Glenside. There were 3 separate pages of documents in their complaint.

The first page ran to 9 paragraphs and purported to be a précis of my remarks at the Establishment sub-committee on 11th March 1966.

The second part was that part signed by my 5 consultant associates. It presented 5 paragraphs of complaints demanding a cessation "of observations which could be interpreted as actual or implied criticism of the competence or character of medical colleagues." It demanded that my responsibilities be confined to my beds and units only and that I should be reminded of my position and accordingly not attend meetings of the Hospital Management Committee and its sub-committees and should not receive the agenda and minutes of meetings since controversies could largely be avoided by use of recognised machinery and by discussion with the Board's Officers and the elected officers of the hospital group.

The third component of the consultants presentation to the Chairman consisted of 10 paragraphs designed to demonstrate that "Dr Early has no statutory position at the H.M.C.", that his attendance caused embarrassment at the Medical Advisory Committee, that he had no constitutional rights to receive agendas and amongst other things he had the opportunity of commenting on policy other than in matters which concerned him. The document which ran to 13 paragraphs ended thus: " The consultants are requesting that he is not now accorded any privilege that they do not enjoy, that he should not attend meetings in a non-constitutional role nor receive any of the documents that they do not receive. The existing state of affairs is causing unhappiness and friction and making it impossible to plan medical work and future developments of the Hospital Group."

Copies of these documents were sent to me by Dr Westwater on 4th April 1966 with the information that they had been submitted to Mr English, Chairman R.H.B. when the Medical Superintendent and Consultants called on him on 28th March. I had not seen them when I myself by invitation visited the Board's office to meet the Chairman on 28th March and had no knowledge of their existence until received through the post on 4th April. My interview with the Chairman was more formal than I anticipated. I explained my point of view.

When I had time to consider in detail the contents of Dr. Westwater's letter, I wrote to him on 13th April 1966 explaining that my contribution to the Establishment sub-committee meeting on 11th March was made after repeated urging from Professor Neale, having resisted his insistence as long as I could in order to avoid raking over the ashes of old controversies. I rejected the contents of the joint consultants document.

I heard no more of the matter.

The Establishment Committee on 11th March 1966 again failed to grasp the staffing nettle and things continued as before.

On 29th November 1967, three weeks after the retirement of Dr Hemphill, Dr.Westwater wrote to the Hospital Management Committee indicating that Dr.Valentine would henceforth be working full-time in Glenside, Dr.Leitch part-time. He added that the next consultant, when appointed would provide additional sessions in Glenside. I voluntarily withdrew from the H.M.C. in December 1967.

At last, after a decade of vacillation the Board had made a decision, a weak-kneed one but better than none. It lasted until the Regional Survey of 1972 laid a more comprehensive plan for reorganisation of the Regional Psychiatric services

But fundamental change was in the air. Parliamentary discussion of the reorganisation of Local Government, of the Social Services and of the National Health Service promised a fresh start to end the muddles of the past. These services were to be brought closely together with administrative structures designed to promote co-operation. The Bills were to be introduced contemporaneously and to go on the Statute Book at the same time in 1972. This was not accomplished but that is another story.

The incidents chronicled in this chapter have been reluctantly related in the belief that their recital is necessary to the understanding of the Fishponds story. They sullied the hospital atmosphere for 2 decades, but with a knowledge of this background progress of the hospital may be more clearly understood.

Early Days in the N.H.S

In 1947, when the first shock of reorganisation had passed, we realised that the categories of patients allotted to us were those which we would anyhow have expected to admit to treat and to care for. Once these responsibilities were complied with there was nothing to preclude the admission of other classes of patients.

Compliance with our admission responsibility was facilitated by the establishment of a regular consultant service to the Observation Wards (Sec.20 of the Lunacy Act) in Stapleton Hospital. This enabled us to exercise some control over this large and increasing source of admissions. By invitation, we established a service to the visiting magistrate by which means the old problem of unloading unsuitable patients on to the mental hospital was partially controlled. It was possible to direct to the mental hospital those patients only who would benefit from psychiatric care and treatment, whilst arranging alternative management for the others who mainly suffered from the illnesses of old age, more suitably treated by the burgeoning speciality of Geriatrics. Thus the complaint by generations of mental hospital superintendents of unsuitable admissions, was partially overcome.

Furthermore there was a tacit agreement with the local Constabulary that persons who came to their attention, who appeared to be mentally ill, would be referred to the Duly Authorised Officer (D.A.O.) for advice and for disposal if appropriate, rather than that they (the police) should detain them or exercise their right to issue an order for admission under Section 20 of the Lunacy Act. Most mentally ill patients thus presented were kept out of the legal system and a useful mainly non-contentious service provided. When Mental Health Act of 1959 superseded the Lunacy Act, the ward ceased to have a function was handed over to Dr Nicholas, the psychogeriatrician, and became a psycho-geriatric assessment unit.

The forties ended in uncertainty. Under the National Health Service the hospital management committee chaired by Alderman Burgess gave the wind of change an acceptable direction. Initially there was often a wish to retain old fashioned practices, e.g. by appointing additional staff to provide services which were rapidly becoming out-dated. They appointed two confectionery bakers to provide on site provision of confectionery for the patients. Usually their decisions tended to be liberal. They decreed the end of the lavish luncheons which used to be separately served to Committee Members and invited them to partake of their meals with hoi polloi in the hospital canteen. They wished all of their employees to have the privilege of Mental Health Officers with regard to conditions of employment and superannuation but the Ministry of Health disagreed. They concurred willingly in serious spending on staff and equipment for new departments such as research and electroencephalography.

Sometimes the changes had unhappy effects as in the case of long term resident patient who for years had successfully managed the patients' shop. The new administrative correctness required that professional business supervision be provided. The patent was asked to resign to make way for a paid shopkeeper. His small stipend was continued but his loss of status led to relapse into deep depression, a condition from which he had been free for several years. He never recovered. He later committed suicide.

The fifties were born in discontent as far as Fishponds was concerned although this is not reflected in John L. Davis' history (1861-1961). However once sufficient clinical freedom was achieved the pace of development quickened. The problem of pulmonary tuberculosis was controlled but the twin horrors of overcrowding and idleness persisted.

Overcrowding continued to be a major problem. On August 17th 1945 there were 1257 patients in residence. In 1951 the HMC agreed to a maximum of 1185 beds. A survey suggested that there should be a reduction to 872 and recommendations concerning all the ward facilities including the kitchens and sanitary facilities were accepted. The plan was supported by the nursing staff and by the Group Engineer. The Committee explained that there were no funds to implement it. When Mrs A. D. Field became Chairman in 1953, she pressed for the division of the large wards and plans were made to this end so that instead of 4 wards each of which housed 110 – 115 patients, there would be 8 wards, 4 with 40 – 45 and 4 with 65 – 70 patients in each, luxury by comparison. Although for a long time nothing took place to bring these plans to fruition, the fact that the problem was again being considered and that some minor modifications were made in other wards such as the extension of the veranda on the female admission ward, gave hope for the future.

Increasing pressure on admissions led to the inevitable accumulation of long-stay patients until the introduction of the Phenothiazine drugs in the early fifties. Even then pressure on beds continued. In 1957 an attempt was made to provide additional space for the aged by the acquisition of Northwoods, a private mental hospital, situated about five miles from Fishponds. Built in 1838 it had 150 beds; it functioned increasingly sluggishly as a private hospital until 1956 when it was taken off the list of approved mental hospitals because of shortage of nurses. This beautiful building and grounds were bought by a local builder who offered the property to the Regional Hospital Board. Discussion with the Matron and Medical Superintendent Fishponds was hopeful. In February 1957 the Mental Health committee of the Board gave approval in principle to purchase and on the 5th of February the Medical Superintendent indicated that the acquisition should be urgently dealt with like a military exercise. By February 18th he had changed his mind, in spite of which the Hospital Management Committee requested the Regional Board to take preliminary steps to buy the property. In due course the Regional Board made an offer which the owner considered to be inadequate and the matter ended there.

In 1951, 12 Grove Road, Redland, which had been used as a residence for 30 long-stay lady patients, was re-organised as a Day Hospital by Dr Stanley Smith Consultant Psychiatrist of Barrow Hospital and Dr Karl Aron who had trained at the Marlborough Street Day Hospital with Dr Joshua Bierer. It was one of the earliest provincial Day Hospitals. The service functioned under a senior non-consultant doctor, initially Dr Aron and later Dr Tony Flood. They undertook the day to day supervision of patient care at the request of consultant colleagues. Day to day staffing consisted of a senior non-consultant doctor a training grade doctor, full-time psychiatric nurses, nursing assistants and occupational therapists. Follow-up out-patients clinics, individual and group psychotherapy, out-patient electroencephalography and ECT were performed there. The hospital was available to all practising consultants and was attended by approximately 30 patients daily. Its sudden closure for redecoration in 1960 left a large number of patients without treatment or support and necessitated the immediate opening of a day service in Fishponds. This developed into the busy Glenside Therapeutic Day Centre, under the care of Dr P. E. Early. Its establishment was facilitated by the availability of nursing staff released by the temporary closure of the Grove Road Day Hospital.

Initially the Glenside Centre was established in the basement of Prichard Clinic and later moved to a free-standing wooden building. Attendance varied from 40 – 50 patients per day. Up to 1983 it served the needs mainly of ageing psychiatric patients whom it supported as part of the Department of Social Psychiatry.

Domiciliary visits (DV) in the patients' own home by consultants with GPs at their request became available in 1948. In the absence of adequate out-patient services the requests for DV's grew to overwhelming proportions. The numbers eased off as general hospital out-patient departments opened: Southmead in 1950, Frenchay in 1952 but they in their turn were rapidly oversubscribed as were requests for advice on in-patients in these hospitals and in their satellite hospitals Cossham, Wendover, Clevedon, Almondsbury and Berkeley. Psychiatric sessions in GP surgeries were established in the early sixties.

In his Centenary Commentary, Laurie Davis described many major and minor occurrences concerned mainly with domestic advances.

The allocation of £96,000 from the Ministry of Health Department's "Mental Million" – a considerable sum in 1955 – provided new accommodation for female patients when the 85 bedded Prichard Clinic was officially opened by the Minister of Health, Mr R. H. Turton in 1956. The Commissioners correctly predicted that it would be used other than for the aged. It was immediately used to "decant" patients to allow the evacuation of wards for decoration and it later became a mixed admission unit.

The central kitchen and the Dining Hall in Fishponds were gutted by fire in 1950 and at the time of refurbishment, heated food trolleys were introduced. They could not reach the first floor wards until lifts were installed in 1952 in which year the first Catering Officer was appointed and refrigeration reached most of the wards. In this year, too, the Ministry of Health dietician visited the hospital and her recommendations brought improvements in the quality and presentation of meals and were followed by the gradual up-grading of ward kitchens over the next 5 years. Dietwise, the per diem allowance of finance for food in the mental health service was but two-thirds of the general hospital allocation. However, food and catering services improved and meal times began to take on a more normal look. Tables seating 4 gradually replaced the large bare refectory table. Tea came from individual pots, sugar in separate bowls, milk in separate jugs no longer from an urn with sugar and milk already added. Condiments appeared on the table and the tin mug the universal drinking vessel disappeared.

Many other, minor, events are recorded throughout the decade:– the sale of the clock tower bells in 1951, the arrival of central television in 1952 and its extension to all wards by 1954, the formation of the League of Friends at a public meeting in the University of Bristol in 1956.

The Church roof was in trouble in the same year. The building itself nearly succumbed but was saved by the hospital works department directed by its master-builder foreman Tom Bromwich. It re-opened in 1958.

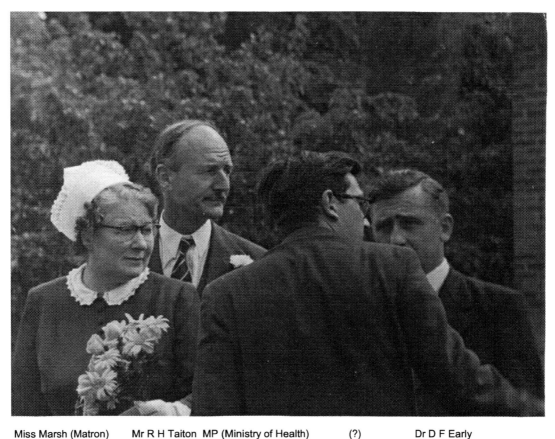

Miss Marsh (Matron)   Mr R H Taiton MP (Ministry of Health)   (?)   Dr D F Early

Figure 54 Opening of Prichard Clinic

The first issue of the Nail, the hospital magazine in 1958 proved to be too ambitious and it was replaced by a weekly roneo-typed sheet *"The Glensider"* in 1969. This successful newspaper survived the 1974 hospital take over up to 1991. It is the main mirror of the denouement of the hospital and is dealt with in a separate chapter.

Pigs which often had honourable mention as food and money producers were wiped out by swine fever in 1958 and so made their exit after a performance which lasted 97 years. Recalling the smells and the yearly infestation by swarms of summer flies, they were not universally mourned.

The new water tower built in 1950, absorbed the entire steel allocation for the West Country mental hospitals for that year. The increased and more consistent supply of water, allowed for many improvements in laundry and domestic use. Communal bathing ceased. The bathroom was converted into an occupation therapy department and later to industrial therapy. The hospital laundry service was noticeably better and it became possible to introduce small domestic laundry on the female wards. "A very kindly measure much appreciated by many," said the Board of Control. Shirts and underclothes began to be personalised in a remodelled and re-equipped laundry department which benefited from conversion of the boilers to liquid fuel in 1953.

Patients who relied on the hospital for clothing still got a raw deal. When quality shirts, underclothing and nightwear were provided, they tended soon to disappear so that institutional standards rapidly returned. Some progress was made in 1954 when suits were sent out for dry-cleaning thus avoiding the familiar scarecrow look of the laundered suit. Real progress had to await the earning of real money by patients later in the decade.

As the decade progressed the standard of life in hospital was improving. Most of the wards had opened their doors. In 1957, two members of the Hospital Management Committee Miss Keen, a retired nurse and Mrs Fields, the Committee Chairman recorded in their visitation report that they were depressed by the inactivity on the wards which they had visited and they plaintively suggested as on so many times before that the provision of hand-work might brighten things up. Paid work was introduced into hospital as a therapy in October 1957. Two Hospital Management Committee members, Cpt. Makepeace and Mrs Korner (later Chairman) wrote in the Visitors book in October 1960: 'Found a wonderful spirit of enthusiasm and a much higher morale. Everyone is working'.

The General Nursing Council in their third visit accompanied by the Regional Nursing Officer, Miss Adams on 9th November 1959 referred to the considerable alterations which had taken place since the first visit in 1951. The four largest wards each of which held between 110 and 115 had been divided into eight smaller wards. Four lifts had been installed. A covered way had joined the wards so that communication did not pass through ward space. Extensive redecoration and partial re-furnishing were recorded. The kitchen and the laundry had been newly equipped. This visitation recorded continued overcrowding on the sick and infirmary wards but concluded that "it was a pleasure to go into the wards and departments and to find the high standard of care and interest maintained throughout the hospital."

In the midst of the busy events of the late 50's, there occurred a catastrophe of a kind most distressing to patients and staff and to the Community at large. A dual child murder burst upon the scene, a nightmare at any time but awful if even remotely associated with a mental hospital.

At 7.30pm on June 20th 1957, June (7) and Royston (5) Sheasby were seen walking by the River Frome in Stapleton, Bristol. They failed to return home and in spite of a widespread search, they were not seen again. On July 1st, 11 days later their small bodies were found in shallow graves in the Grove near Snuff Mills a wooded part of the estate of Bristol Mental

Hospital. Decomposition made it impossible to establish if there had been sexual interference.

Emotion in the City ran high and Local and National papers were not slow in indicating the proximity of the mental hospital to the gruesome find. Banner headlines in the Bristol Evening Post asked "Is this monster still prowling while the children of Bristol are at play?" followed by: "Are there among the big population of mental institutions in the area patients whose medical records indicate them as people who may suddenly lose all self control?" These questions were supported on the front page by a separate paragraph in emphasised type: "Patients Checked. Already Bristol detectives may be on the path to answering some of the questions posed by parents. They are planning a personal check on hundreds of patients in Bristol Mental Hospitals. Preparations for the big scale enquiry into the background of many patients were formulated to-day. Detectives spent four hours with Mr J Davis, Secretary of Bristol Mental Hospitals Management Committee."

Thus began for staff and patients probably the blackest month in the history of the hospital, which became the headquarters of a thorough and determined police investigation. It was made clear by us to the police that there was a total unity of interest between them and the hospital patients and that during their investigations all their reasonable demands were met without demur.

The Chief Detective Superintendent took little part in the day to day interrogation which responsibility fell mainly on Chief Detective Inspector Jesse Pane and Chief Detective Inspector George Aston and their teams. They asked that medical supervision be provided whilst they interviewed patients. This was agreed and no patient was interrogated without the support of a medical or nursing officer known to him. The police behaved with commendable courtesy and restraint. The going was tough for them also, but only once did one of their number overstep the bounds of correctness and he was removed from patient interrogation. The enquiry was conducted with consummate skill and hopes were high that the perpetrator of the horrible act would be brought to trial.

No hospital patient was seriously considered as a suspect nor was sufficiently firm evidence uncovered against any other person who was questioned. No one was charged and the case came to an unsatisfactory and uneasy end.

In 1964, Dr A Hyett Williams of Oakwood Hospital, Maidstone published in the medical journal the Lancet, details of a prisoner who had committed suicide in Derby prison. Dr Williams recorded that before his death this prisoner had admitted to the murder of two children. The Home Secretary took exception to Dr Hyett Williams' publication of the case and he had an uncomfortable time.

The Sheasby case was one of only two double child murders in England this century up to that date so that the case of the dead prisoner, if his admission were true, might have been able to shed light on the case. We waited until the furore had died down and we wrote to Dr Williams on December 10th 1964 to ask him if he would kindly consider writing a letter to the medical press to the effect that the prisoner about whom he wrote was neither in-patient nor out-patient in a psychiatric or mental hospital at the time he committed the murders. It was pointed out that we were involved in the investigation of the murders and that since the bodies of the children were found on the hospital estate, the suspicion lingered in some quarters that one of our patients may have been involved. He replied promptly that he understood our views but because of all the trouble over the case, he had forwarded our letter to the Medical Defence Union for advice. In due course, one month later he replied "I would like to inform you that the Medical Defence Union have strongly advised me against any communication with the medical press."

We fared no better with Chief Inspector Pane. On 19th March 1994 he said that he did not wish to discuss the case. Detective Inspector Aston died some years ago.

The cloud has never been authoritatively lifted.

But life went on, the new decade mirrored the enthusiasm which was fuelled by the opening of the factory of the Industrial Therapy Organisation in March 1960. This movement designed to help toward open employment and towards open living was largely initiated and developed by the hospital staff, mainly nursing, who now felt part of the main stream of psychiatry and were enthusiastic and encouraged by the local, national and international comings and goings which surrounded their daily activities. The extra hospital development brought a new dimension of experience with exposure to new exciting ideas not only to patients but the staff of all departments who met a wide range of business and professional people. The nursing staff acquired new skills cross-fertilised by their industrial fellow workers with whom they worked side by side. Their contribution was invaluable. They had to get on with their own skills since there were neither professional social workers nor psychologists working in Fishponds at that time.

The development of hospital services followed contemporary trends. Prichard Clinic was at first used as a decanting ward and later became a busy mixed sex admission unit. Discrete male and female admission wards were also maintained for those patients to whom mixed living was distasteful or even abhorrent. Interchange of male and female staff was introduced generally in the hospital in 1962. About this time to we admitted mothers with their babies to Prichard Clinic until such time as a unit for their special care was opened in Barrow Hospital.

Patient visiting was formally liberalised and was encouraged at any reasonable time with precautions to ensure the relatives were advised not to arrive unannounced if his or her relative spent a large proportion of time outside the hospital.

Hospital social life was organised more and more by the patients themselves. The League of Friends and the H.M.C. gifted a club house to staff and patients. The patients club was very active. Glenside Museum has inherited a notable collection of gramophone records which belonged to the social club having been bequeathed to them by a resident.

Extra hospital practice continued to grow. Out-patient departments in Southmead and in Frenchay General Hospital were always busy as were requests for in-patient consultations in these and other general hospitals. GP consultations were established in Southmead Health Centre. In 1962 Derek Russell-Davis, Prof was appointed to the Chair of Mental Health in Bristol University. He established an under graduate teaching unit in Glenside which although it took little part in the corporate life of the hospital it added an exciting element in the teaching of undergraduates.

The burden of domicilary consultations lessened as out-patient clinics developed. A consultant appointment to the Medical Officer of Health (Dr Woffinden) widened relationships with the Mental Health Department of the Local Authority. Day attendance at The Day Hospital in Glenside recorded an attendance of 2362 patients in 1962.

Centenary celebrations of 1961 were marked by a highly successful exhibition between 4th and 24th May 1961 at the Royal West of England Academy Bristol. The subject was 'Bristol in the Evolution of Mental Health 1696 –1961'. The 100 years of Glenside was almost lost in the wider consideration given to other local services. The H.M.C. celebrated the centenary by joining the League of Friends in the purchase of a social centre. A request was made for the provision of religious facilities for the Roman Catholic patients in the new social centre. This was agreed and Mass continued to be said there until access to the hospital church of England was requested and granted in 1969.

John L Davis, the hospital secretary produced a historical account of the first 100 years from the annual reports of the Visiting Committee. The 20 foot high wall which separated the hospital from Manor Park Hospital was reduced to a height of 4 feet. It was jocularly suggested that this wall should now carry a plaque stating that its height was reduced in commemoration of the hospital centenary! At least the threat of being sent "over the wall" was reduced.

In 1962 again the male nursing staff was honoured by the award of MBE to Louis Walker the Nurse manager of ITO and later that year Alfred Baldwin, the Chief Male Nurse was appointed to the newly established Hospital Advisory Service. Charge Nurse Leslie Law was appointed Social and Group Organiser of the long term rehabilitation in-patient unit, and prepared many men and women for discharge. It did not survive Mr Law's resignation in 1967.

In 1963 John Chamberlain the new Chairman of the Hospital Management Committee was informed by the Regional Board that they had included in their capital programme for 1963-68 the building of a unit at Glenside for the treatment of patients suffering from alcoholism. After months of discussion it was reported that the August meeting of the Hospital Management Committee (1963) that an in-patient unit exclusively for such treatment was not advisable. The hospital minutes referred to a memo in which the suggestion was discussed but this memo was missing, so the arguments deployed are not known.

A joint appointment of a Psychiatric Social Worker (P.S.W.) by the Local Authority and the Hospital Management Committee was agreed in February 1964. Mrs Hellfrich was appointed to this post but the balance of the requirements of each authority had not been sufficiently carefully explored. The appointment failed.

In May 1965 a request by the University for residential facilities at Glenside was acceded to. Living in students started work and lived upstairs A nurse training unit which had begun in May 1967 was completed in March 1969 and received students. There was two-way secondment of student nurses between Glenside, Southmead Hospital and Frenchay Hospital.

The Mental Health Act 1959 abolished the word mental from the title of psychiatric hospitals. After a long search and tedious debate 'Glenside' was the best that could be found.

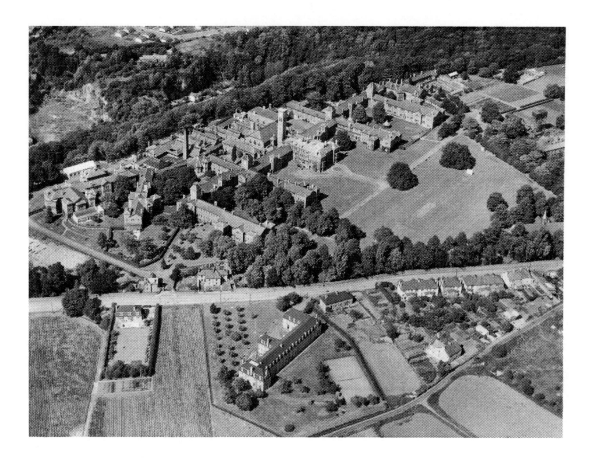

Figure 55 Bristol Mental Hospital 1954

Medical Supt. House left foreground; Nurses Home middle foreground

The Story of I.T.O - A Job to Do .

The collapse of the Research Department was a bitter disappointment. At the time there were, however, major compensatory medical and social advances. The introduction of active psychotropic drugs was heralded by Chlorpromazine ("Largactil") in 1952. It was in general use by 1954. Many others followed, each capable to a greater or lesser extent of controlling or relieving some of the more disturbing symptoms of mental illness. They were joined by the anti-depressants when Imipramine Hydrochloride ("Tofranil") was introduced to hospital trial in 1959 and became universally available in the following year. These soon began to augment the social changes already in train and gave a realistic possibility of discharge to long-stay patients, which in turn demanded consideration of suitable extra-hospital facilities for these patients and for such of those who could be treated without the necessity of admission to hospital.

In 1956 the Commissioners of the Board of Control echoed the obvious - that there was "a failure of effective rehabilitation within the hospital" and they reiterated the long held view that in-patient care should be therapeutic, not custodial. Idleness had always been identified as the most malignant obstacle to patients' independence. Occupation Therapy departments lacked trained staff and few of the residents were considered capable of serious work in hospital departments. Mostly, the best that could be hoped for was "ward work" a euphemism usually applied by the Sister or Charge Nurse to pulling a "bumper" around a polished floor or wielding an ineffective duster, devices to ensure that patients would be on the "pay roll" and would not be entirely penniless. The more efficient individuals worked for a slightly higher financial reward in one of the maintenance departments – the gardens, the kitchen, the laundry, the sewing room. The Commissioners talked about the re-establishment of the habit of work. They may even have understood, although they never said so, that O.T as established would never succeed in accomplishing this aim and that employment in the hospital maintenance departments, the most realistic work available, was as exploitative as it was therapeutic. They offered no solution when they intoned in 1957 that "this is a major task and if it is to be effective entails re-organisation of the entire hospital."

In that year (1957), there were 137,000 patients resident in the mental hospitals of England and Wales. Hospital wards housing 100 to 120 patients were not unusual. Conditions within them were abysmal for patients and staff alike. Neither the local authorities nor the Ministry of Labour nor the hospital services provided or were likely to provide the means to improve their condition.

Many attempts were made over the years to introduce into hospital real work for real pay. These were often briefly successful but there was no long-term commercial break-through. Baker's work in Banstead Hospital in 1956 (Note on Life of J. P. Turley) confirmed our local experience that many patients were capable of productive work but with N.H.S. red-tape and with neither capital, nor ideas, nor commercial nous, we found it impossible to set up our own commercial organisation.

Idleness remained the norm until Dr Owen E. L. Sampson introduced to us Mr John Turley the Managing Director of the Tallon Pen Co. an industry to manufacture ballpoint pens which depended mainly on out-workers. Dr Sampson was a Bristol GP who took a major interest in community affairs. He was the first Chairman of Glenside Hospital League of Friends. He was Chairman of Bedminster (Bristol) Rotary Club and later National Chairman. He was currently in the process of selling his house to Mr Turley. Dr Sampson knew that we had had occasional success and had been seeking for many years, a way of establishing realistic work for patients in the hospital. John Turley had previous experience in trying to help with the employment of the Local Authority's protégés with learning difficulties but his efforts had foundered on the inability of the supervisory staff to achieve

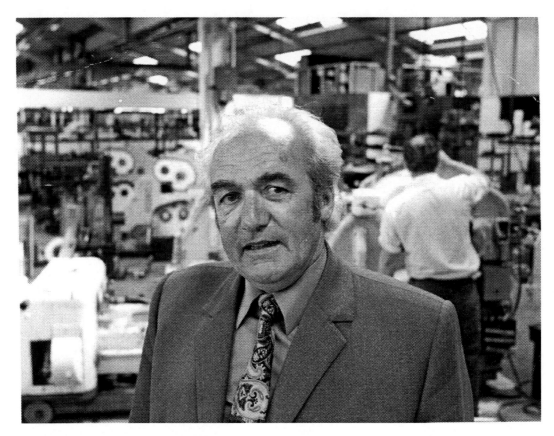

Figure 56 Mr John P. Turley   M.B.E.

consistent quality control. He was a philanthropist of great compassion but his commercial interests were incompatible with consistent loss making work.

He was invited to visit the Occupational Therapy Department (O.T.) of Fishponds hospital. In spite of the apparent pointlessness of much of the activity which he saw, he agreed that many of the patients there were capable of productive work and reckoned that they would improve with proper training and incentives.

He agreed to put ball-point pen making into the hospital on a trial basis on the same state of pay as were currently paid to his own out-workers. He was unwilling to repeat his previous experiences of untrained supervisors and suggested that his firm provide industrial surveillance. This was readily accepted. He initially appointed as supervisor Mr Fred Parry, one of his senior foremen, an experienced, understanding and tolerant middle-aged man. He supervised the first couple of months in the hospital shops and when he returned to his parent factory Tallon employees continued routine industrial supervision of patients side by side with the hospital nurses.

We believed that at last we had a serious chance to break into industry, a view shared by the Matron, Mrs Golden and the Chief Male Nurse, Mr Alfred Baldwin. As a factory we occupied part of disused night nurses' accommodation. The maintenance department found suitable furniture and fittings mainly discarded from wards during their modernisation. Louis Walker a senior Charge Nurse was under treatment for hypertension and the Chief Male Nurse thought that he needed relief from his onerous job as joint Charge Nurse in a 115-bedded ward. He was asked to organise the nursing supervision.

In November 1957, the pen components arrived and work began.

The first 7 patients had been well chosen. They were paid by output, 2/6d [12.5p] for assembling a gross of Tallon's "Wagtail" pens. Not royal pay but enough to set the tongues wagging. As they gathered experience patients could earn 10/- [50p] per day and more. The highest payment to patients working in hospital maintenance departments was 10/- per week and soon the holders of these sinecures asked how it came about that patients less efficient than they and lower down the pecking order, could earn so much for a change!

The trial period was successful – so much so that when Mr Parry returned to the factory, quality control of new contracts was completely carried out in the hospital. The wards buzzed with excitement. The Ward Sisters and Charge Nurses agreed, occasionally reluctantly, to review with their M.O. the work potential of their patients and to place them on a list in order of potential industrial efficiency. They also agreed not to try to prevent any patient wishing to do so, from going to work in the Industrial Therapy Department (ITD). They faced a dilemma. What would happen if all the ward workers chose industry? It was jocularly suggested by one Charge Nurse that one or two of his less energetic colleagues might have to do some work.

The Hospital Management Committee was informed that the staff structure of the hospital would change as patients deserted maintenance departments to work in I.T.D. They accepted this calmly. Initially they charged 10% of I.T. department income for the use of hospital facilities but this deduction was soon quietly forgotten and they were in the vanguard of support.

Success was cumulative and by the end of 1958, one third of the patient population of the hospital – 380 patients – was employed in the I.T.D. Supervisory staff was not hard to find amongst the nurses, although some of them opted out because they considered that "working for an industrialist" was not a nursing duty. Mostly they and all other branches of the staff were convinced that there was no element of patient exploitation and that the proper location of professionals was wherever the patient needed assistance and guidance. Working locations multiplied, the male Occupational Therapy Department, a disused general bathroom and a large chicken hut were utilised and eventually when busy the dining hall, part time. The maintenance staff were always able to find furniture.

N.H.S. rules did not cover this development. Outside hospital at that time up to £1-19-11d [£1.99] per week could be earned without loss of NHS benefits but there were no specific rules covering our situation, so we paid patients the amount which they earned on piece work, sometimes up to £4 per week. Owen Simpson let the cat out of the bag when triumphantly relating the success of the scheme to a Rotarian luncheon in Town. National Insurance Officials reacted promptly and weekly payment had to be limited to £1-19-11d. Thereafter, by agreement, amounts earned by individual patients in excess of this, were held in a fund to boost the earnings of less able patients.

Prior to the introduction of industry only 3 patients earned "wages" of £2 to £3 per week from hospital sources. The next most useful of the higher paid helpers received 10/- [50p] per week and they soon changed their jobs for a 400% increase in industry. It was to the great credit of Ward Sisters and of Charge Nurses that they did nothing to prevent their 'star' patient helpers from moving to I.T.D. And move they did. Some of the long-stayers soon started to be discharged from hospital. For the less active there was a tendency to settle down in hospital on a relatively high income.

The hospital staff clearly understood that the earning of small sums of money by their own effort by long-unemployed people was an invitation and an incentive to progress, if possible to a living wage. At this stage it was not absolutely clear how this could be accomplished but suspicions of exploitation were allayed by the patently open method of management which showed that patients were the only possible beneficiaries of the work. The introduction of paid work as a form of therapy in 1957 acted as a revolutionary stimulant to activity and produced an immediate and visible change amongst men and women alike. It obviously raised the standard of living, dressing improved, socialising became more cordial as did contact with relatives where they were in contact. The number of wholly unemployed patients fell to about one third of patients surveyed in 1960.

The earnings of patients demonstrate an increasing earning potential:

from: ANNUAL REPORT ITO 1962

		1957	1958	1959	1960	1961
No. of patients in hospital		1200	1172	1169	1147	1122
Hospital Allowances		£6820	£5980	£6194	£7082	£8685
Industrial Earnings	In Hospital	—	£3731	£8706	£10043	£11510
	I.T.O. and Sheltered Workshop	—	—	—	£7943	£11743
	Open Employment	—	—	—	£3750	£4368
Patient Earnings		£6820	£9711	£14900	£28818	£36306

Figure 57 Patient Earnings - from I.T.O. annual report 1962

In 1959 John Turley had obtained the lease of a disused Church of England school near to his factory which he intended to use as a collecting centre for the Tallon ballpoint pen out-workers. Knowing how we wanted an outside step for rehabilitation, he offered places in the old school where patients could go from hospital for employment by the day. It was suggested to him that the establishment there of a factory for the use of patients working on a piecework basis would be even more useful. He accepted this suggestion and took the initiative in the formation of a company appropriate to our needs. The discussions for its establishment started late in 1959. Sir William Grant, Chairman of the West of England Branch of the Engineering and Allied Employers Federation became Chairman of a new company called the Industrial Therapy Organisation (Bristol) Ltd (I.T.O.). The Board was made up of representatives of the Churches, Industry, Trade Unions, the Local Authority and the Medical Profession and adopted as its motto "Through Work to Health." We claimed 3 Bishops on the Board, the Bishop of Bristol, the Bishop of Clifton and the President of the Free Church Council until the latter said that we could refer to him as we wished but not as a bishop! The Lord Mayor was amongst the first Board members, with the Regional Secretary of the Transport & General Workers Union – Ron Nethercott and Professor Woffinden the Medical Officer of Health of Bristol.

There was publicised concern from the Bristol Trades Council. They too, feared patient exploitation but their fears were set to rest at a Press Conference, where the patency of the financial arrangements reassured them.

I.T.O. was registered as a company limited by guarantee in January 1960 and opened for business on March 7th 1960 in the old St Silas School in York Street, St Philip's Marsh, Bristol. On the opening day 60 patients came by bus from Glenside Hospital and started work. There were a further 10 men direct from their own homes. The factory was staffed by supervisors seconded from the firms for whom we were working and by nursing staff from the hospital. The H.M.C. cut away all sorts of red tape to enable this major early community development when they accepted the view that the nurses' duty was where the patient was and that supervision in the factory was as essential as on the ward.

The factory settled down quietly and quickly but Union suspicion simmered until finally assured by Frank Cousins, the General Secretary of the Transport and General Workers Union, when he visited I.T.O. later in March 1960. He recommended Trade Unionists to

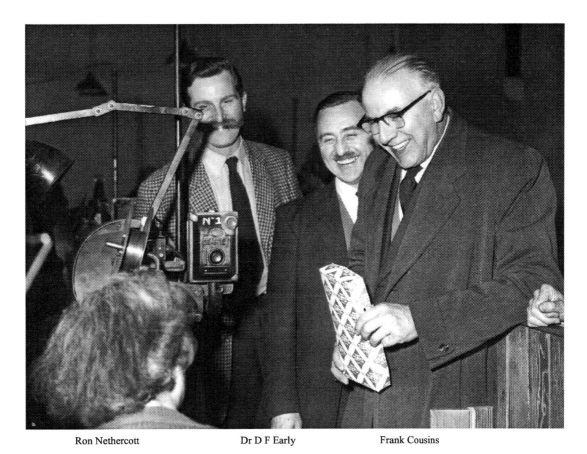

| Ron Nethercott | Dr D F Early | Frank Cousins |

Figure 58 Frank Cousins visiting I.T.O March 1960

support initiatives like I.T.O. and he allayed the fear that patients were being exploited or that they were in any danger of being so in an organisation such as I.T.O.

Following a visit by Professor John Wing and the late Dr Douglas Bennett, they too were able to assure medical colleagues that I.T.O. was a genuine effort to help with the hitherto apparently insurmountable problem of economic rehabilitation for the "chronic" hospital population.

I.T.O. was regarded as stage 2 in work rehabilitation for the long hospitalised patient on the way to stage 3, work in open industry or commerce. Industry was prosperous, industries were numerous and locally controlled, industrialists were generous, it was immediately possible to arrange with them either to employ I.T.O. rehabilitees individually or in groups in their factories or on a training or trial basis. This became known as the Labour Loan Scheme and in the early days was the main source of jobs on the open market. Patients thus employed were usually taken permanently on to the company pay roll.

In November 1960 a car wash project was launched which provided paid work for 14 patients bringing "chronic" patients face to face with the general public, a financially profitable venture and socially successful.

Patient referrals from hospitals (Mental and Subnormal) and from the Community (Local Authority and GPs) were numerous and hopeful. At the end of the first year the slow movers began to accumulate and as a partial answer to this problem. I.T.O. established a Sheltered Workshop, in which the then Ministry of Labour made good 75% of financial losses up to a maximum of £150 per place per annum.

The establishment of the Sheltered Workshop was agreed in 1961 in discussion in the Ministry of Labour HQ in London. This was attended by 12 or more Whitehall Civil servants representing the Ministry of Labour, Social Security, National Assistance and

National Insurance amongst others. This was an awesome meeting for the administrative unsophisticates of I.T.O. but the Sheltered Workshop was agreed for up to 25 places, later increased to 50. The Sheltered Workshop approach was always a second best option. The Ministry of Labour insisted that this was an end point in rehabilitation and that those who achieved it were in full time work. It was therefore not considered by them as a step on the way to open employment but I.T.O. used it as such.

The two years 1960 and 1961, were successful and saw 55 patients become wage earners in open industry and 51 in "sheltered work", some after very long periods of unemployment. The two-year follow up was encouraging. A film of the initiative, *The Right to Work*, was sponsored by Smith Kline and French, had a wide national and international distribution and won the British Medical Association (BMA) Bronze film award medal 1961.

The Labour Loan scheme having proved successful, I.T.O. suggested to the Ministry of Labour that the terms of support to individuals in sheltered workshops could be applied to groups of workers in open industry who were stable in work but who had not yet reached full earning capacity. We sought to negotiate the application of the sheltered workers subsidy to groups of our patients working in open industry under our aegis for independent employers.

Discussion on this topic was comparatively short and not without humour. When the Ministry agreed to meet our representatives, I.T.O expressed the wish to have a delegation comparable in quality and numbers to theirs. In view of the experience with the Sheltered Workshop discussion in 1961 it was proposed in the I.T.O. delegation should consist of the Lord Mayor of Bristol, the Bishop of Bristol, the Bishop of Clifton and the Chairman of the Free Church Council, the Regional Secretary of the Transport and General Union, the Chairman of the Engineering and Allied Employers and so on up to a number matching the Ministry delegation. This suggestion was met with a good humoured response that it would be better to avoid a rugby team and that 4 on each side would suffice on this occasion! And so it was. Our Managing Director John Turley, David Sladen, newly appointed Regional Chairman of the Engineering and Allied Employers Federation West of England Branch, Ron Nethercott Regional Secretary of the Transport and General Workers Union and I, met Mr Stewart of the Ministry of Labour and three colleagues in September 1962. Their arguments that the employers would not agree to our proposals were refuted by David Sladen and that trade unions would adamantly oppose were rebutted by Ron Nethercott. On the grounds that it amounted to the subsidisation of wages, the civil servants opposed us, all except Mr Stewart who said that he could see no argument that would debar such a scheme and accepted it for further consideration. Many months passed during which time, we were later told, it was brought to national employers and trade union organisations. Eventually in July 1963 we were informed that our scheme had been accepted. It was hedged around with conditions some of which seemed almost impossible to fulfil e.g. that patients should be fit to leave hospital and should have accommodation available, that groups must consist of 10 or more patients employed under direct professional supervision in open factory conditions. This virtually precluded the employment of men as the work was unsuitable for them. This was the subject of repeated negotiation by John Turley with the Ministry. Eventually it was agreed that 10 patients working in smaller groups or at individual tasks could be supervised peripatetically. So a group of one was successfully established! Many sheltered placement workers went on to open employment although the Ministry did not see this as the purpose of the scheme. Later "Sheltered" Placements were adopted by the Department as the "Enclave Scheme." This obnoxious term was later dropped in favour of "Sheltered Industrial Groups."

This scheme which the Department initially opposed vigorously on the grounds that it amounted to the subsidisation of wages has now become national policy with repercussions far beyond the field of Psychiatry.

The 1974 re-organisation of the Health Service saw mental hospitals under the management of the general hospital, which knew little about the problems of Psychiatry and showed scant inclination to enquire into them. Nursing support for I.T.O. by Glenside Hospital (now run for Frenchay District Authority by the administrators of Frenchay General Hospital) continued precariously and it became evident that the arrangements made by the old H.M.C. were not going to be honoured by the new Hospital Trusts who could see no logic in their District budget covering the expenses of patients who were possibly chargeable to other districts. This argument was far removed from the needs and interests of long-stay hospital patients whose district of origin (if any was recorded) related possibly to five, ten, twenty or more years previously. The districts, in turn were subdivided with professional direction from psychiatrists with increasingly narrow sub-specialities and with little emphasis on the "chronic" services. The Nursing link – so important to I.T.O. finally snapped in September 1991 when without discussion or notice the occasional nursing visit from Bristol District (Barrow Hospital) ceased.

In 1992, a survey of I.T.O. patients by the Medical Registrar of one of the more recently appointed Consultants with a responsibility for rehabilitation proved only to be a delineation of district chargeability, which addressed neither clinical nor social needs. I.T.O conducted its own survey the Annual Medical Report 1993 and considered that all 90 patients seen were in need of support. There was no other organisation, which was prepared to provide a service for them.

The numbers of hospital referrals to ITO has gone down year by year, which reduction has been compensated for by the increased referrals neither from the Health Authority nor the Local Authority, nor from any other source. The fall has continued and therefore the number of employees goes down. In 1994 the Board of I.T.O. agreed that they themselves would employ nursing and occupational therapy expertise to attempt to re-establish a multi-disciplinary training plan for the personal requirements of each referral. This has not been accomplished and the Thirty-seventh annual medical report of I.T.O commented on this and concluded that there being no medical element left in I.T.O.'s programme an annual medical report no longer served any useful purpose. It was therefore discontinued. There is now no on-going professional help from day to day nor any assessment of referrals or discharges.

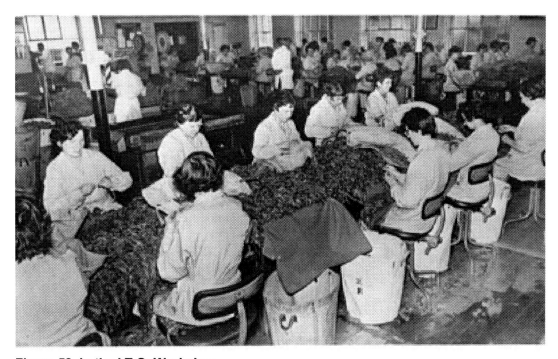

Figure 59 In the I.T.O. Workshop

INDUSTRIAL THERAPY ORGANISATION (BRISTOL) LTD.

MEDICAL REPORT
for year ended 31st December 1992

Mr. Chairman

I have the honour to present my thirty-third Annual Medical Report on I.T.O.

As was the case last year, there has been little medical input during the year.

On the 1st December 1992 I reported to you the result of a survey which I carried out on worker-patients during the previous month:

SURVEY - November 1992:

In I.T.O. I surveyed 56 worker patients - 51 male, 5 female.
Their age varied from 22 to 76 years.
Their time at I.T.O. from 1 to 29 years.
Their abilities varied greatly: at least 8 are not suitable for I.T.O. and are deriving little benefit from attending.

Classification under headings: (1) the source of referral when known - (2) the present district of residence - (3) diagnosis.

(1) SOURCE OF REFERRAL		(2) RESIDENT IN POSTAL DISTRICTS
Farleigh Hospital	15 Males	3(x7), 4(x3), 6(4), 7, 8, 18
Barrow Hospital	2 Females	8, 14
	10 Males	2, 3(x2), 4, 5, 8, 13 (Clevedon)
Glenside Hospital	1 Female	16
	3 Males	16, 6, 8
Purdown, Stoke Park and Hanham Hall	6 Males	3, 5(x2), 8, 15, (Yate)
Burden	2 Males	16, 18
Southmead	2 Males	7, 8

The remaining 13 patients all show clear evidence of involvement of the subnormality services e.g. resident in group homes, have spent time in the Blackhorse or Bush TC, educated in Florence Brown school, etc..

SOURCE OF REFERRAL		RESIDENT IN POSTAL DISTRICTS
Subnormality	2 Females	5, 15
Service	11 Males	3(x2), 4(x5), 5, 6, 11, 13

I classified the patients under the diagnostic heading of subnormality or mental illness. This does not mean that the condition is active nor that medical treatment is currently necessary nor that the conditions are mutually exclusive:

Of the women	3	Mental Illness
	2	Subnormality
Of the males	13	Mental Illness
	38	Subnormality

5 patients suffer from idiopathic epilepsy

These (very) raw figures are presented to you with a hope that I.T.O.'s future functions and funding will be illuminated by them.

I have found only two patients who expressed positive dissatisfaction with I.T.O. In answer to the question "what do you feel about I.T.O.?", a surprising number of enthusiastic replies were received, e.g. "Lovely", "I enjoy it", "They've been marvellous", "It's a therapy, and a couple of pounds a week". Most were less enthusiastic.

I considered all the worker-patients surveyed to be in need of support. I am not aware of any other organisation which is prepared to carry this burden. I do not consider that it should be I.T.O.'s task to decide which authority is responsible for this task.

In the Sheltered Workshop and Sheltered Groups there are 23 people, 21 men, 2 women. These are employees of I.T.O. and supported by the Government's Employment Service. I have not considered their characteristics. They are the concern of neither the Health Authority nor of the Local Authority except insofar as the continuation of these services depends on the continuation of I.T.O.

As far as the year 1992 is concerned, at the year's end we employed:

A) I.T.O. Workshop: 66 worker-patients, 59 men and 7 women. During 1992, 4 people were taken on and 5 were discharged, a reduction of 1 patient.

B) Sheltered Placements: 3 employed, unchanged from last year.

C) Sheltered Workshop: 21 employed, 19 men and 2 women, unchanged from last year.

Total number under care at I.T.O. on December 31st 1992 was therefore 90, 1 less than on December 31st 1991.

Figure 60 One of the last annual medical reports for I.T.O. 1962

At its first meeting of I.T.O. in 1960 it was explained to the directors that they were founding a "suicidal" organisation in that their purpose was to provide stage 2 of industrial and commercial rehabilitation for the patients of Glenside Hospital. Success would mean that there was no longer any necessity for the service. Glenside Hospital is no more. It might have been better for I.T.O. to have withdrawn from the fray when its primary purpose was accomplished. Now it flounders in the avaricious, ill-organised seas of the Hospital Service and Community Care. It is still the largest facility of its kind in Bristol, and at the time of writing the largest industrial employer in a district which once housed the Imperial Tobacco Company. It has neither medical nor nursing, nor psychological nor social work support from statutory authorities, although it needs to survive if only for the sake of its 80 – 90 workers and its staff.

The Hospital Patient Surveys 1960 - 1990

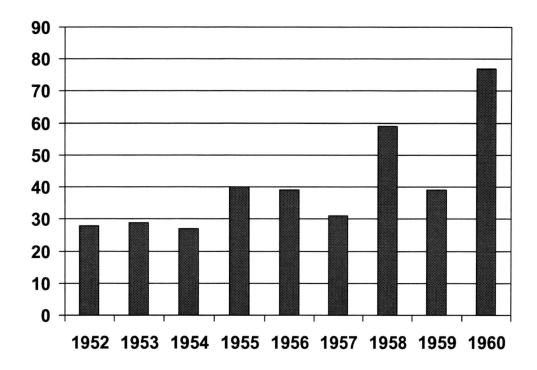

Figure 61 Number of patients who had been in hospital for over a year, discharged 1952 - 1960

There was a dramatic increase in the discharge rate of long-stay patients in the late fifties. The introduction of phenothiazines undoubtedly played their part but was unlikely to have brought about the 100% increase, which occurred in 1958, the year that industry was introduced into the hospital or the three fold increase in 1960, the year during which the Industrial Therapy Organisation started work.

The downward national trend was analysed by Tooth & Brook in 1959 and they concluded that if the then trend continued the mental hospital population would fall nationally by 2% per annum in succeeding years.

At the Annual General Meeting of the National Association for Mental Health in 1959, Enoch Powell, then Minister of Health, latched on to these conclusions. Out of the blue and with neither discussion nor consultation with professionals, he used this untested statistic to announce a plan for the closure of 40% of mental hospital beds within 10 years.

To test the predictions of Tooth and Brook, and to asses the possible needs of our patients Dr.Brian Cooper (later Professor of Psychiatry Heidleburg University) and I undertook in 1961 a survey of the resident patient population in Glenside hospital. We surveyed 1012 patients who on the day of the survey had been continuously resident in the hospital for three months or more. We wished to define the mental state of each patient with particular reference to their outside employment possibilities and their accommodation needs. A schedule of 34 items was completed on each patient. Our information was obtained from case notes, by discussion with nursing staff, by reference to central hospital records and by personal interview such as necessary to complete the schedule.

	Male (%)	Female (%)	Total (%)
Psychiatric Care	288 (63.5)	270 (48.2)	**558 (55.1)**
Geriatric Care	21 (4.6)	62 (11.1)	**83 (8.2)**
Supervised After-care	118 (26.1)	136 (24.3)	**254 (25.1)**
Unsupervised After-care	17 (3.8)	50 (4.0)	**67 (6.6)**
No Special Arrangements required	9 (2)	41 (7.3)	**50 (4.9)**
Total	**453**	**559**	**1012**

Figure 62 First Hospital Survey 1961

Using the same schedule, the hospital population was subsequently surveyed every five years over the next thirty years, seven times in all up to 1990. In 30 years the total population fell 72% from 1012 to 294, a decline of 2.4% per year.

This series of surveys was described by Catherine O'Driscoll (The TAPS Project) as the best known repeated survey in the UK of a single hospital primarily aimed to focus on the accommodation and employment needs of patients. They also documented other patient characteristics and changes which took place in the last thirty years of the life of an underprivileged Victorian mental hospital.

The population became more aged each five years: 22% of men and 43% of women in 1960 were aged 65 and over, the corresponding figures in 1990 were 51% and 70%, with only 16% under 45 years of age.

Possibly the most dramatic finding of 1960, was the number of patients who were no longer in need of hospital care but who were so institutionalised that they could not and or did not actively seek to, live outside hospital. Three hundred and seventy-one patients, 37% of those surveyed, needed no special hospital arrangements and could be catered for in supervised or unsupervised after-care accommodation. This figure as a proportion of residents varied little over the next 30 years in spite of efforts to counteract it. In 1970 the corresponding figures were 288 (38%); in 1980, 114 (27%); in 1990, 119 (41%). These figures, consistently reported, were not catered for by the Social Services. One wonders what became of them.

Survey after survey confirmed the friendlessness which showed no improvement over the years. This was the saddest and a significant finding. It rang alarm bells for community psychiatry, a warning of the possibility of isolation being worse outside than inside the hospital. In 1960, two hundred and one (201) in-patients had no known relatives or friends and were seldom or never visited; in 1970 one hundred and forty three (143); in 1975 one hundred and ninety five (195) and in 1980, two hundred and seventy-nine (279).

Amongst the factors involved in this phenomenon were unmarried status, length of stay in hospital and old age. Ford and his colleagues described the situation as "scandalous." He concluded that community care is surely a sham in the absence of the necessary infrastructure of service and financial supports. In 1990, four years before the hospital closure Eastley and her colleagues described the figure of two hundred and fifteen friendless in-patients (215) as "staggering." Only 12 out of 158 patients in hospital 5 years or more were visited, "and equally disturbing" only 14 of those in hospital from three months to two years. It was considered that many of the patients "could enjoy a better quality of life in the community but discharged without appropriate provision of locally based services would be sentencing them to an isolated impoverished existence... Their quality of life should not be allowed to deteriorate as the mental hospital is run down and resources are withdrawn."

This clarion has sounded down the years. Twenty years ago Nicholas and I wrote that the local authorities' track record before 1948 was one of providing a sordid hospital service for the mentally ill and that there were few developments since then or indeed since 1959 or since 1974 which would give hope for a future in their hands. Hospitals close. Loneliness, isolation and rejection are still rife with few appropriate activities for the shy and withdrawn.

As the years rolled by the hospital population aged. In 1990 more than half of the men and nearly three-quarters of the women were over 65 years old (20% and 43% in 1960). The number detained was rising; a secure unit – Fromeside Clinic had been opened and the total number detained approached the 1970 level.

The honeymoon period of economic rehabilitation had passed. Only four patients worked outside the hospital and only 17 attended the Integrated Rehabilitation Workshops, thirty six worked in hospital departments or did ward chores leaving "a massive 237 patients with no work." This fall in numbers from 349 workers (37%) in 1964 was related not only to national industrial decline and the reduced "chronic" hospital population but also to their increasing age, their lack of social support. By 1980 paid work therapy in hospital was increasingly kept afloat by day patients. Its virtual cessation by 1985 was mourned by Ford and his colleagues as being to the detriment of more than one third of the hospital population who occupied impoverished ward environments with minimal staff and who suffered personal poverty, no longer able to supplement their income from Industrial Therapy.

In 1961, we advised Professor Woffinden, the Medical Officer of Health for Bristol that he could immediately, safely plan for accommodation for 90 clients. We recommended to him that about 30 in-patients would require no nursing supervision. If individual resettlement proved impossible we recommended that these patients could be cared for in groups not exceeding 15 residents and that a further two supervised hostels each of no more than 30 places could be planned with confidence. Over the next 30 years, one fifteen bedded single sex hostel was provided by the Local Authority. It succumbed to economy cuts, in the early seventies one of the first victims of local authority economies.

After the Local Government Reorganisation of 1972 Local Authority made no realistic attempt to provide our categories of clients. The Bristol Industrial Therapy Housing Association (BITHA) was formed in 1962 with the intention of providing affordable accommodation and was able to indicate some possible approaches.

Joint funding was unsuccessfully explored in 1976 and again by Ford and his colleagues in 1987. He reported an unsuccessful attempt to involve joint funding in the provision of appropriate accommodation and concluded that projects from social service departments and voluntary agencies could probably deal with only a small proportion of the problem. He was proved correct.

In 1961, we viewed Tooth and Brook with anxiety, wondering what was to be the fate of our 371 patients who did not require continuing treatment. The Mental Health Act 1959 prescribed extra-hospital living but as usual failed to provide the necessary finance to allow the Local Authority or the Ministry of Labour or the Hospital Service to prepare for or to provide the most basic requirements of community living – as job to do and place to live. I.T.O. tried to establish a step by step approach to the former. A place to live remained a challenge.

The Story of I.T.O   A Place to Live

In the 1960 survey there were 371 in-patients who no longer required hospital accommodation. Each succeeding count brought to light many in the same category for whom no appropriate living conditions were available in the community. In 1959 Government funds were said to have been provided by way of an increase in the Local Authority's block grant but little or no new accommodation appeared on the ground. There was nowhere to live and no funds available for the psychiatric patient continuously and unnecessarily hospitalised.

Historically "Living in the community" was the traditional fate of the psychiatric patient from time immemorial. Little welcome was ever to be found there. Relief came with the Lunacy Act of 1845 and the mandatory provision of asylum beds by local authorities. Before this date only Bethlem and a few places like St Peters Hospital, Bristol offered residential help to the pauper lunatic whilst a range of private madhouses provided services which ranged from the luxurious to the cruelly sordid.

The ideals underlying the development of the Victorian Asylum were wise and philanthropic but parsimony and self-interest soon led to their fall into disrepute. The humane movement in Psychiatry intended that hospitals should be small so as to provide a personal service. As early as 1862, the second year of operation of Fishponds hospital, the Chairman of the Asylum Visiting Committee had discovered that the neighbouring asylums could care for many more patients with the same number of staff as he employed. Fishponds, which was intended to treat not more than 250 patients, had grown to 1,100 by 1910. From its opening the ever increasing admission rate caused the hospital to stumble from one overcrowding crisis to another.

Mental hospitals and hospitals for 'Mental Defectives' had nationally garnered nearly 200,000 beds by 1948. In-patient costs were cut to the bone, as their numbers continued to rise.

Rapid social change and the introduction of active drugs in the early fifties meant that many of the socially disruptive symptoms of mental illness, particularly of schizophrenia, could be relieved. Hospital admission could then be more frequently avoided, the length of in-patient stay became shorter and the discharge of 'chronic' patients was often a realistic possibility

The sudden unexpected announcement by Enoch Powell that he agreed with the predictions of Tooth & Brook and that he proposed that mental hospital beds should be reduced by 40% in 10 years caused dismay in hospital circles where there was no confidence that funds would be produced to replace the facilities for this large number of patients. Powell maintained that the block grant to Local Authorities had been increased to provide the necessary range of community developments under the Mental Health Act 1959. This was not evident to the mental health services in Bristol. Almost unanimously hospital professional staffs understood that the day of the 'isolated, majestic, imperious and daunting' mental hospitals (as described by Enoch Powell) were finished but few could see what would take their place. Nor were they given much help in this regard. One Ministry paper followed the other, often contradictory in their recommendations and prognostications.

We always had difficulty in re-settling socially unsupported patients in the community. Before Prichard House was built in 1956 we made a request that a couple of standard Council houses should be built in the hospital grounds to aid in social re-training. At that time Council houses cost £1,200 to build and we felt that £2,400 from the proposed £90,000 (approx) allocated (as Bristol's share of the "Mental Million") to the building of Prichard House would cause an insignificant reduction of its bed complement. The suggestion was not accepted by the Regional Hospital Board. When I.T.O. was up and running and increasing numbers of "chronic" patients were in work, there was no sign of provision of outside living accommodation.

In 1960, negotiations took place between Fishponds H.M.C. and the Bristol Corporation Housing Authority to build 6 standard Council houses on the hospital estate. The H.M.C., the Local Authority and the R.H.B. agreed to the proposal but opposition from Whitehall delayed the project (as they did so many times in the future). When this was overcome the local political situation had changed and negotiations had to be re-opened. Geological and climatic complications then beset the project. Finally the contractor had financial problems so that the occupation of these houses was delayed until 1965.

By this time we had formed a Housing Association – the Bristol Industrial Therapy Housing Association (B.I.T.H.A.) and in March 1965 had bought and renovated the Vale Hotel a private hotel in a residential district. For this the Transport and General Workers Union (T.G.W.U.) lent us £10,000 on generous terms which enabled us to buy and partially to renovate the premises, and to install central heating. Having established a Housing Association, the H.M.C. requested B.I.T.H.A. to take over the tenancy of the Council houses, which was agreed.

In 1970, the Industrial Therapy Housing Association acquired Belgrave House, a large Victorian house on the Downs which belonged to Southmead General Hospital and had served as their preliminary Nurse Training School. Southmead Hospital Management Committee readily agreed to our suggestion that they allocated the house to B.I.T.H.A. for the use of discharged patients. They accordingly informed the Regional Hospital Board who agreed the offer but felt obliged to inform the Department of Health. This evoked the usual

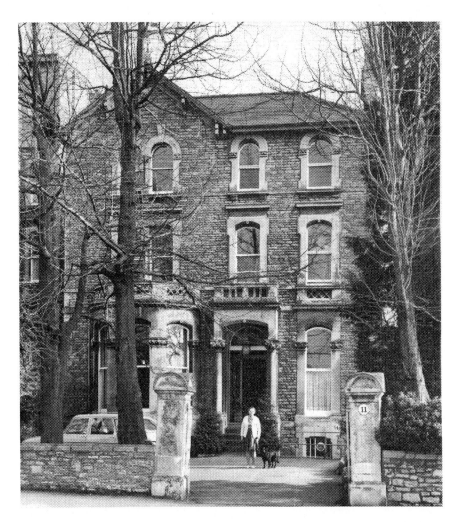

Figure 63 Belgrave House

110

negative response that the Department could not let Government property to a voluntary organisation. It appeared that that was that. However Richard Crossman, the then Secretary of State was visiting Bristol on political business and at our invitation dined with John Turley our Managing Director, Eric Buston our P.R.O. and myself. He listened with expletive disbelief to our problem and less than one month later agreed to lease the property at a nominal rental to B.I.T.H.A. – a development which he referred to as "something achieved!" This house situated on Bristol Downs provided accommodation for 31 residents on 5 floors.

In 1972 the house next door to the Vale Hotel was offered for sale to the Association by the owner who ran a nearby hotel. We appealed for funds to Dr Woffenden the M.O.H, who referred our request for financial support to the Social Services Committee. They bought the house, gave us tenancy and when finally purchased they transferred ownership to B.I.T.H.A.

Conforming to the norms of the time, these developments provided residential places for 89 residents and were run economically to a high standard. This did not mean that they were the cheap option sought by the politicians, but demonstrated that there was a large group of mental hospital in-patients who could achieve normal living conditions outside hospital without too much fuss.

Opposition from bureaucracy is difficult to foil although victories can be achieved in minor encounters, e.g. when preparing to furnish the Blackberry Hill houses, we asked the patients in the hospital Industrial Therapy Department (I.T.D.) to work one extra hour per day to contribute toward this object. With a few refusals they agreed. The Hospital Management Committee (H.M.C.) agreed to hold this money for us in their funds. When the time came to acquire carpets, furniture and bedding the H.M.C. prepared to release our money. Before doing so they dutifully informed the Regional Hospital Board who agreed but dutifully informed the Department of Health who promptly said "No. No funds from hospital sources to a voluntary organisation." This arrogant misrepresentation of the facts was overcome by the H.M.C. buying the necessary furniture and equipment and transferring it to B.I.T.H.A. on permanent loan.

Architect's plans were prepared for the provision of about 50 places in a variety of dwellings to be used as flatlets, houses (group houses), bed sitters and some larger houses (or smaller ones joined together) to provide unsupervised and supervised accommodation – to be built without frills and to represent the type of accommodation which would normally be available on the open market and which would allow for individual choice. We suggested that these be built with joint Care Planning funds and that the Management be handed to B.I.T.H.A. who would be responsible for the tenancies in all respects.

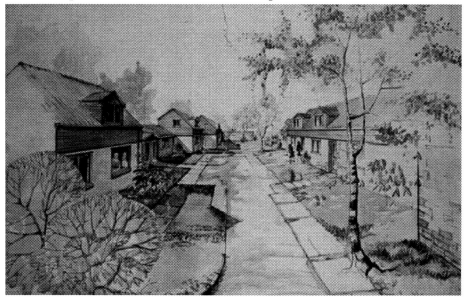

Figure 64 Proposed Trial Campus Layout

This we called the Campus Project for the domestic resettlement of psychiatric patients designed for training, trial and demonstration of ability of patients prior to final discharge so that they could make an informed choice as to their domestic needs and requirements and be seen to be capable of achieving them.

By discharging up to 50 "chronic" patients, 2 wards in the hospital could be closed. This would release for other work --including supervision of rehabilitation – 20 nurses, which we thought was more than adequate to staff the scheme.

The hospital staff was enthusiastic but not the local authority whose Director of Social Services did not see his responsibility as covering "in-between cases" and not the Area Community Physician who "liked the idea" but suggested that a loan from the Housing Committee would be more appropriate. The plan failed to proceed with Joint Care funding. The Director of Social Services said "It is a difficult scheme to process as it involves 3 statutory services and a voluntary organisation." Perhaps this was not unconnected with the fact that the Local Authority (Social Services) needed £200,000 to pay off the debt on a recently erected Training Centre for subnormal patients.

B.I.T.H.A. thought that the Campus Project was a good scheme and sought financial support elsewhere. We approached the Housing Corporation who expressed appreciation of B.I.T.H.A.'s previous housing record and set aside money for the project. Negotiations opened but unfortunately we were faced with the same bureaucrats, who had considered our application under Joint Care Planning. The only difference now being that B.I.T.H.A. was no longer competing for Joint Care funds. We hoped therefore for their support. The Director of Social Services wished us well but said he could not provide social workers to supervise it but that he would not oppose the project. The Area Medical Officer said that this was now a new scheme, a residential, not a training scheme, which he could not approve unless the District Health Authority agreed to the new circumstances. The whole whirligig started again. The Frenchay District Psychiatric Advisory Committee again agreed to the scheme. Provisional approval was once again given to the sale of the site for the Campus development and the Frenchay District Health Authority uninvited took over the negotiations with the Housing Corporation whose Regional Controller (Mr Morgan) supported our project and wrote

> May I say how interested and impressed we were with the pioneering work B.I.T.H.A. has clearly been undertaking in the field of community care for ex-psychiatric patients. It is apparent that your organisation had appreciated the importance of this field of endeavour long before it became fashionable to espouse it, and, more importantly you have been able to put many of your ideas into practice...

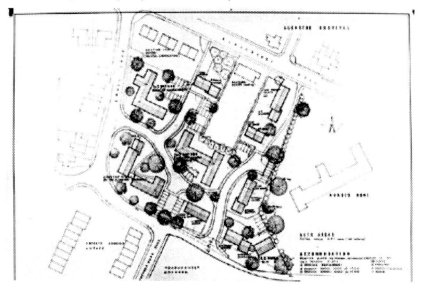

Figure 65 Plan of proposed housing - Nurses home is to right, Blackberry Hill passes across top of plan.

Mr Morgan expressed that "the emphasis must be on reaching agreement with tenant on the best type of housing to meet his needs" and agreed that to decide this, a licence could be issued for a probationary period to see if this tenant could cope with his/her chosen accommodation. In this he accepted and understood the "trial" purpose of the campus development better than any of the statutory authorities.

The National Health Service reorganisation placed the management of Glenside Hospital and estate in the hands of Frenchay Health District in which the hospital is situated. They were ignorant of psychiatric matters and of I.T.O.'s and B.I.T.H.O.'s contributions to rehabilitation. Wires got crossed from time to time and following one particularly disagreeable meeting of I.T.O. with Local Authority and health officers in March 1979, negotiations almost broke down. The Housing Corporation remained supportive and even suggested an extension of the scheme which entailed the development of housing on a larger area of land with dispersement of the I.T.O. units which could be expanded or diminished as required.
Mr Turley and B.I.T.H.A.'s architects suggested that this larger scheme be carried forward by the Knightstone Housing Association who from there on undertook the negotiations on B.I.T.H.A.'s behalf.

We were not kept very closely in touch until our architects heard from Raymond Jones, the Frenchay District Administrator in October 1980. It seemed as if the negotiations had got out of hand. A copy of Mr Jones' letter to the architects was sent to 9 other people but ominously not to B.I.T.H.A: "Reservations are still being expressed... but the District Management view is that they need not prevent the scheme going ahead... The medical staff (of Glenside) generally supported the proposal but Dr Dabbs and Dr Babiker have asked for more time to consider related aspects... no decision has been taken." On 29th July 1980 Babiker wrote "I can see no reason why we should not give our approval to the scheme..." and asked that his views be communicated to the Director of Psychiatry.

As far as B.I.T.H.A. was concerned there was silence then until information was sought in 1983. It was disconcerting then to be informed that a firm decision was made by the Fishponds Sector Management Team on 14th April 1982 "that the land surrounding Clonora (the proposed site) should not be sold to the Knightstone Housing Association as it was felt that the proposed housing development would not be of benefit to Glenside Hospital." This letter was dated 14th June 1983. Dr. Nicholas, Senior Consultant at Glenside recalls no such decision being made by the Glenside medical staff committee.

Our original proposal was in May 1976, 7 years earlier. There was no further communication.

As late as 8th January 1987 the Baroness Trumpington Joint Under Secretary of State at the Department of Health and Social Security wrote to the then Director of the National Schizophrenia Fellowship: "The fundamental point is that the Government does not have a policy which is geared primarily to the run-down and closure of mental illness hospitals."
The Hospital service (A.H.A.) said it was the Local Authorities responsibility. Social Services said it was the Housing Committee's. The Housing Authority said it was the hospitals' and so the project died to the benefit of the Health Authority.

It was a cause for anger to us but not of surprise that the hospital land was sold for private housing development in 1990 for £2,500,000. Glenside derived no benefit from this rapacious transaction. Nor did the psychiatric service in general, for whose benefit the land was acquired more than 100 years previously. The Campus Project was intended for the use of the citizens of Bristol most of whom benefited not at all by this particular sale of the family silver.
BITHA, renamed the 'John Turley Memorial Housing Association' in 1992, continues to provide accommodation for the psychiatrically ill.

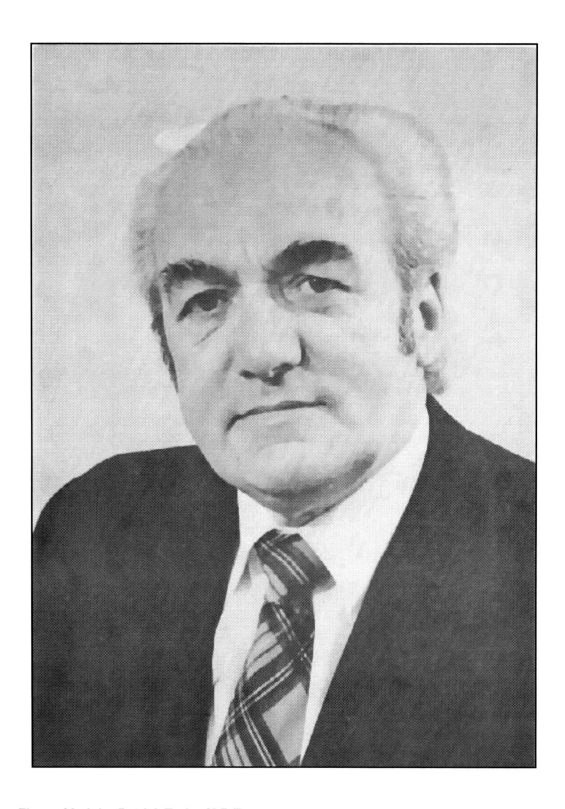

Figure 66 John Patrick Turley M.B.E.

JOHN PATRICK TURLEY M.B.E.

Managing Director, Industrial Therapy Organisation (Bristol) Ltd 1960
Industrial Therapy Housing Association 1962

John was born in Glasgow in 1919, the son of a merchant seaman. The eldest of a large family, at the age of 16 he emigrated to London and worked for Swan Fountain Pens. He married Kathleen in 1941 and they had four children, one son and three daughters. John died on 22nd May 1990.

In the 1939-1945 war he served in the Merchant Navy as a 2nd engineer, and survived many hazardous voyages. After the war he returned to Swan pens and having attended night school to study new industrial and management techniques, was put in charge of production planning. He later became Works Manager at Waterman pen factory, Leicester, from whence he joined Bristol Repetition in 1954 as General Manager.

Bristol Repetition was a small private company whose worker-owner saw the potential of growth in ballpoint pen refills. John Turley built up the company, which later included the making and marketing of ballpoint pens under the name of Tallon. He put assembly work of these pens into a work unit at Glenside Hospital, Bristol in 1957.

The success of this venture led to the birth of the Industrial Therapy Organisation in Bristol in 1960. John Turley was the master builder. The association between ITO and Glenside Hospital in the treatment of mental illness enjoyed a national and international reputation over many years. He held that Government should support and expand employment opportunities – particularly sheltered work. He believed that employment was nature's best physician and was essential to human happiness.

In 1964 the ownership of Bristol Repetition and of Tallon Limited changed hands. John found his job advertised by the new owners before he knew he had been dismissed. Within 9 weeks he had made a fresh start with his own company, Auto-Precision Limited, having in that space of time travelled round the country, contacted potential customers and suppliers and arranged to lease anew factory. He then located, inspected and negotiated the purchase of plant and machinery, and engaged the first staff.

From beginning in 1964, without capital and with one small factory and 5 employees, John Turley's business grew until, by 1980, he owned a group of companies with 1,500 employees and seven factories located in various parts of the country. During this time he remained firmly committed to the Industrial Therapy Organisation.

John Turley travelled widely in his industrial work and made contact with psychiatric rehabilitative factories and workshops as far afield as New York, Moscow and Hong Kong. His publications included The Right to Earn a Living, Work as a Factor in Mental Health, and Economic After Care.

John Turley also played a leading role in 1962, by establishing the Bristol Industrial Therapy Housing Association, whose assets were merged with ITO in 1987. Now, in 1995 to commemorate his work, these assets are transferred to the new John Turley Memorial Trust.

Reorganisation   Regional Survey 1971 –72

At the end of the sixties Parliament produced three major bills which proposed the reorganisation of Local Government, of the Social Services and of the National Health Service. These bills *inter alia* promised co-operation between the services in place of the existing muddle which had grown up over the decades. The three services were to have 'administrative co-terminosity' which was to make joint decisions possible. It was proposed that the bills be introduced contemporaneously. A change of Government prevented the bills reaching the statute book together. Only the bill for the reorganisation of the Social Services became law in 1972, so that the other two had to await modification by the incoming Tory Government.

Secrecy and the uncertainty dogged the development of plans. In spite of this, late in 1970, the Board requested me, as Chairman of the Regional Psychiatric Advisory Committee to carry out a survey of the psychiatric services and to produce proposals for the development of mental illness services in the Region. This was organised under the administrative guidance of Dr Bruce Telford, Medical Officer of the R.H.B. (Psychiatry) whose service to Psychiatry has not been adequately acknowledged. It was undertaken during the period December 1970 to December 1971.

The plan for the National Health Service was announced by the Government in March 1971 and proposed 'to unify the National Health Service and the Health Authorities outside local Government'. Details were not revealed. Information was hard to come by. The South Western Regional Hospital Board was not permitted to inform the Glenside Hospital Management Committee of the future plans for the group. At an extraordinary general meeting of the Committee on April 27th 1971, the Chairman was able to divulge his information only to the committee members and then only in confidence i.e. in secret. Many discussions were taking place on the future pattern of the service but they proceeded with little information so that Health Service integration could not be sensibly discussed nor could new relationships with the Social Services.

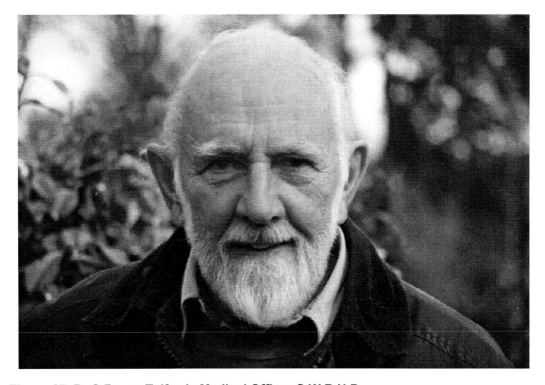

Figure 67 Dr S Bruce Telford, Medical Officer S.W.R.H.B.

Our Review Committee was asked to consider and to report on the long term needs and plans for mental disorder including mental illness and mental handicap, interim and short term needs and requirements, the medical establishment, the nursing establishment, Local Authority provision for mental illness and mental handicap, such as hostels and any other special needs or developments already planned or likely to be required. As time went on mental handicap was dropped from our remit.

The core members of the Committee (Dr Doherty - Child Psychiatrist, Gloucester and Cheltenham; Dr Jancar - Consultant Psychiatrist, Subnormality, Stoke Park Hospital Bristol; Dr Regester - Medical Officer of Health, Gloucester; Dr Early - Consultant Psychiatrist (Adult) Bristol; Dr Bruce Telford - Medical Officer (Psychiatry) R.H.B. and Mr Fox – Nursing Officer R.H.B.) represented adult and child psychiatry, subnormality and public health (as these specialities were then called) and the regional nursing service. Local consultants, public health doctors, nurses and social services managers and representatives of other disciplines joined the discussions and sat on the committee from district to district.

The Review of the Regional Services 1972, ran to 92 pages and entailed the visitation of the seven main National Health Service Psychiatric hospitals in the region, North Gloucester clinical area, Bath clinical Area, Bristol clinical area, Tone Vale Hospital (Somerset), Exe Vale group of hospitals, Exeter (Devon) and the West Cornwall group. The United Bristol hospitals (The Teaching group) made its own recommendations as an independent submission. This was incorporated in our final report. The report was presented to the South Western Regional Hospital Board by Dr Telford in January 1973 as 'Proposals for the Development of Mental Illness Services in the South West Region' (Copies of which can be found in Glenside Hospital Museum). It ran to 41 pages, 5 of which referred to Bristol.

Comments in this chapter will relate mainly to the services provided by Glenside Hospital which were considered by a sub committee consisting of Dr Bakker Chairman, Professor Russell-Davis, Dr Jancar and Dr Early. The Committee met on 15th, 17th, 25th & 29th of June and on the 2nd July 1971 and discussed the future of the services for the mentally ill in Bristol Clinical Area.

The Committee had available to them the Report of the Bristol Area Hospital Services Review Sub-committee chaired by Dr Frances Page which had proposed for Bristol three closely integrated District General Hospitals each with provision for the mentally ill. Our Review Committee agreed with long-term aims that there should be comprehensive facilities for mental health services at the three District General Hospitals, Frenchay, Southmead and the United Bristol. In the medium and short term it recommended that Glenside Hospital should continue to serve as a centre for mental illness to which consultants in adult mental illness working in the district should be attached. A continuing function would allow that special units should continue to be developed on the site.
In discussion with Local Authorities we foresaw "little difficulty in arriving at sensible arrangements defining catchment area would be the same for local authority and hospital services."

The Committee based their detailed staffing and accommodation proposals on the figure included in the draft circular on Hospital Services for the Mentally Ill, that a District General Hospital (D.G.H.) serving a population of 250,000 should have 0.5 in-patient beds and 0.65 day places per 1,000 population. The resultant reduction in current bed numbers could be taken as a basis of planning, only on the assumptions that "back up" facilities would consist of special psychiatric units on the mental hospital sites and that there be adequate residential facilities in the community. "There is evidence that this is not being provided. It cannot be stressed too strongly that very many patients remained unnecessarily in hospital because of the absence of suitable community accommodation." The concept of custodial mental illness units was not acceptable. Community accommodation of a domestic nature should be provided by the Hospital services for patients with continuing psychiatric symptoms in Community hospitals, the then current suggestion.

The suggested formula would provide for 400 beds and 515 day places, i.e. 120 beds and 150 day places in each of the three District General Hospital. This would mean the closure of a considerable number of mental hospital beds as these units come into use.

Recommendations for the provision of medical services for Frenchay and Southmead Districts – the Glenside catchment area followed the recommended norms. Each district North East (Frenchay) and North West (Southmead) had a population of approximately 250,000 so that in addition to its in-patient and day-patient accommodation each district would require a complement of 4 whole-time consultants in Adult Mental Illness who between them would conduct 15 out-patient sessions per week. In the short term an in-patient facility of 30 beds with day hospital and out-patient support would be required.

Medical staffing: Each medical team was to be headed by a Consultant Psychiatrist supported by adequate staff. Each Consultant team was to be responsible for a population of almost 60,000 people i.e. 4 teams per district.

Nationally there were 1.5 Consultants per 100,000 population. In the South West Region this figure is 1.37; in Glenside - Barrow group 1.02. We recommended that this should be brought up to the national average as soon as possible.

We recommended:
1. A consultant in N.E. District based on Frenchay and Glenside. Equal interest co-ordination and expansion of day services.
2. A consultant in N.E. District – Frenchay & Glenside to develop further the rehabilitation service.
3. A consultant with an interest in the Elderly in N.W District based on Glenside and Southmead.
4. A consultant in charge of the services for alcoholism and we would hope to encourage a greater involvement of general practitioners in the work of the hospital units.

This brought the number of consultant teams in each of the NE and NW Bristol Districts to four.

As beds fell, Glenside was to continue to provide major "back up" facilities for a number of special units. The occupational and domestic Rehabilitation service were to be developed for up to 200 patients in Glenside for whom it would be possible to plan rehabilitation with the ultimate aim of discharge. An additional consultant team would be required, supported by training and domestic accommodation, both on hospital premises and in the community. Interim and short-term in-patient units at Frenchay and Southmead were urgently recommended with extended Day hospital accommodation. Special facilities for the treatment of alcoholism were to be developed including an additional consultant with appropriate staff and accommodation in the community.

Appointments were made shortly after these recommendations. Consultant Services for Alcoholism came later.

A clear need was stated to develop services for the elderly with one consultant team per district in the first instance. The assessment unit in Manor Park was not functioning effectively because patients could not be placed elsewhere. Local Authority provision and the possibility of establishing day centres at existing Local Authority hostels was to be explored and the extension of voluntary services to be encouraged.

Dr. Crow of the Burden Neurological Institute advised that a Neuro-psychiatric Unit in Bristol could serve an Area or a Regional need providing brain surgery, in-patient treatment of epilepsy plus rehabilitation and aftercare of brain damage. The needs of Child Mental Illness, Electro encephalography and Clinical Psychology were briefly commented on as needing separate consideration.

The review ended with the advice that the presence of two doctors was always needed at electropexy sessions (E.C.T.), one with experience in anaesthetics.

We did not feel competent to make recommendations on the organisation of the Nursing Service. Three nursing divisions each controlled by a Nursing Officer would be necessary, in each of the D.G.H.'s. On the nursing evidence presented to us we recommended centralised training; amalgamation of hospital nursing schools would lead to more comprehensive courses including a stint in the Community.

The complications of the different areas used by each Local Authority were noted. Bristol divided into five social service areas. We ended up with 5 Hospital districts Bristol NE, Bristol NW, Bristol South, Bath and Weston-Super-Mare. Bath later opted for Wiltshire and Weston-Super-Mare was incorporated into Somerset. The 3 Bristol areas had to divide so as to serve 5 social service areas of the City.

The 5 Directors of Social Services with whom we conferred in 1972 and the boundaries within which they operated were not those in post when our report was presented to the Board in 1973. The blandness of our statement that it was felt "that the opportunities for discussion and exchange of views with its Local Authority Officers has been useful and can be regarded as the beginning of an essential dialogue between the services" says it all.

Proposals for the Development of the Mental Illness Services in the South Western Region were presented to the R.H.B. by Dr. Bruce Telford in 1973. They briefly described the present services and the catchment areas then under discussion.

The Board accepted that Mental Illness Units should be provided in Southmead Hospital, Frenchay Hospital and Western-Super-Mare with United Bristol Hospitals who were considering a similar new hospital in South Bristol.

The recommended provision for Avon Health Authority less Bath was to be:

	Beds	Day Places
Southmead	150	200
Frenchay	150	200
Weston-Super-Mare	50	70
United Bristol Hospitals	(BGH 30)150	200 (BGH 40)
	(BRI 120)	(BRI 160)
TOTALS	**500**	**670**

The Timings were:
  Southmead – It is hoped to commence the building of the new mental illness unit at Southmead in October, 1975, with a completion date in December, 1977.
  Frenchay – It was also hoped that this development would commence in October, 1975, with a completion date in June, 1977.
  Weston-Super-Mare – This is due for completion, with its mental illness facilities, in 1978.
  Timings for the development of the Bristol Royal Infirmary were not for our committee's consideration.

The R.H.B.'s recommendations for Glenside were:-
  Glenside and Barrow Hospitals are now reorganising on a catchment area basis and are developing consultant therapeutic teams oriented towards the future District General Hospital catchment areas. Thus when the new units are opened the existing teams will be ready to centre themselves on the District General Hospitals.
  The opening of these new units will allow a reduction in the number of beds at both Glenside and Barrow, but both these hospitals will have to continue to care for long stay patients until alternative accommodation is provided by both Hospital and Local Authority for those who are inappropriately placed in these hospitals, particularly the geriatric and the psychogeriatric patients.

Glenside is likely to continue to provide the long stay requirements for both Southmead and Frenchay and may become a centre for sub-Regional services, i.e. rehabilitation, forensic, alcoholism.

The future turned out differently. Southmead District alone provided a comprehensive psychiatric service with in-patient, day patient, out-patient and community facilities. Frenchay District and South Bristol District, fund holders of the Glenside and Barrow services continued to utilise the old hospital facilities whilst trying to provide the community service which our committee considered to be responsibility of the Local Authorities.

The Final years: The Glensider and the Press

The Glensider proved difficult to establish as a newspaper to chronicle day to day hospital happenings on a regular basis. In March1958 a roneo-printed publication – the Nail – made its first appearance and produced 13 issues up to Winter 1971. Its latter issues were professionally printed and well produced; style and content varied from fair to very good; its Centenary Edition in 1961 was notable. It failed to appear at regular intervals and its "news" was stale before its appearance.

A less ambitious production, *The Glensider* was launched in September 1969. It was edited by Leslie Button, a well known and trusted Assistant Secretary whose interests covered every aspect of hospital life, and was presented as "a news sheet produced in an effort to improve communications between management and staff and to keep all our patients and staff in touch with the happenings in and around Glenside."

And so it did. It immediately attained a wide circulation throughout the hospital and beyond. Les Button edited 200 editions consecutively up to November 1974 when he handed over to Linda Hopkins (later married name Graves) then a senior administration assistant who edited the next 639 editions for 14 years to October 1988. She was then superseded by David Payne who finally "with a certain amount of sadness" put the old lady to bed with edition No. 941 January 1991.

In January 1991 it was replaced by a new look "Health Authority Serving Our Community" news sheet "Focus" which ran through 20 editions under different editors between March 1991 and January 1992. It attended the dying moments of the hospital with a brief paragraph on the 9th January 1992 headed "Glenside's Last Supper" when it was briefly reported that "the recent Staff party Last Supper was a huge success."

The first issue of *The Glensider* described recent hospital ward re-grouping, the provision of a new hospital shop, a new ladies and gents toilet, a new Nurse Training Unit and a promise of many other plans "of which more later." There was a 'Do you know?' article informing the reader that the annual Hospital budget "is now approx 1½ million pounds of which salaries claim approx £940,000," that 650 staff care for 1000 patients, longest serving member of staff Male Nurse Fred Knight, joined in February 1927, the longest stay patient was admitted on 3rd September 1909 – the first patients were admitted in 1861. This issue concluded with a welcome to staff newcomers and a notice of pending farewells and presentations – a regular feature in each edition. This format was continued often in a humorous style during Les Button's supervision; facts were accurate, opinion independent, gossip light hearted and apposite. Linda tended to be more factual but she could not resist a joke at times, as when she suggested that an advert for a temporary guillotine operator required someone to dispose of the increasing number of redundant staff. Some themes recurred year by year; parking problems, increasing difficulty in gathering sufficient news.

It is possible to follow the dismemberment and destruction of Glenside year by year and to trace the hospital mood as it realises that reorganisation is not unequivocally patient or staff friendly.

Morale was high during the late sixties and early seventies so that at times the mood was almost euphoric. Describing progress made during 1970, Les Button writes that "it's certainly the Swinging Seventies as far as Glenside is concerned"; even the staff ball had 600 guests, the largest for years.

Anxiety and doubt about the future were often expressed. The edition of 23rd of March 1972 reported a welcome to Visitors from Local Authorities of Bristol and of Gloucester and which noted the closer relationship between local authorities and hospital services proposed under new and pending legislation whilst expressing doubt about the current view that because an organisation is bigger it is necessarily more effective. "What little experience I have had, has proved the opposite to be true", wrote the Editor. Later Roy Everett, Hospital Secretary, in May 1972 at the A.G.M. of the Association of Hospital Management Committees at Bournmouth questioned whether ex-psychiatric hospital patients were receiving adequate care and attention in the community.

Mrs Korner the Chairman meeting 100 staff in September 1972 was unable to assuage these feelings. The spirit of optimism was soon overshadowed by the word "strike." "Staff complain that they know less of what was happening than in the old days of the bush telegraph." Constructive proposals were promised but senior management knew next to nothing and could not satisfy staff. Gloom at times bordered on despair, not alleviated by a visit by Christopher Thomas the Chairman Designate of Avon Area Health Authority.

But exuberance broke through again and again. "The festive period of Christmas 1973 will rank as one of the best ever in Glenside." Hope revived, but was not consolidated by the Declaration of Intent by the Avon Area Health Authority on January 1st. Glenside was to be managed by Frenchay District. The Chairman was to be Mr Christopher Thomas and the Secretary Mr Brian Thomas. It was stated "that the mists of uncertainty are now lifted." *The Glensider* did not comment that Mr Chris Thomas had been vice-Chairman of the H.M.C. of the United Bristol Hospitals, the teaching hospital, and Mr Brian Thomas its financial officer.

With Mrs Korner, they met the Glenside Staff on 31st January. There were too few questions; the problems were not yet evident except that there was but a small smidgen of democracy in the new service, the Community Health Council, which had few teeth. Worse was to come - the realisation that the Medical Director, Dr Alan Snaith was not acquainted with Psychiatry and that unlike the old Regional Hospital Board the Area Health Authority (A.H.A.) was not required to establish Psychiatric advisory machinery.

On the occasion of the 25th Anniversary of the N.H.S. the Editor prophetically wrote: "I am sure that the vast hierarchical monster to be imposed on us from 1st April 1974 will become an administrative monster and will itself consume many thousands of pounds which could be put to much better use at ward and patient level." Dies Ira – the Hospital Management Committee was dissolved at a meeting on 4th April 1974. Having functioned since 4th July 1948, it quietly accepted its fate, without comment.

In November 1974 Les Button became Administrator of the District Mental Illness Sector and on 21st November he relinquished editorship of *The Glensider* to Linda Hopkins. She was to inform the readers for the next 14 years.

In May 1975, Les became Sector Administrator in the Stoke Park Hospital Group (Learning Difficulties). Glenside was never quite the same again. Before his departure he wrote some memorable leaders in *The Glensider*: on 13th November 1973 'Who's kidding who?'; on 3rd January 1974 'Well 1974 is here' and on 4th July 1974 'The Budgetary Allocations' in which he mused that the bad old days of the past may be looked back on as the good old days.

As Linda Hopkins began her long editorship, one by one the old retired. Norman Kearns Deputy Clerk and Steward and long time Deputy Secretary left in June 1975 after 45 years service. Mr Owen in charge of the Path Lab for 20 years was 'transferred back' to Frenchay and the Fishponds lab closed after 80 + years.

On 6th November 1975, Alec Haslett, the New Administrator took up his post. In February 1983 he became Unit Administrator. In April'86, he was transferred to Manor Park Hospital.

The year 1975 produced 32 issues only of *The Glensider*. What little comment there was betokened the increase in influence of the National Union of Public Employees (N.U.P.E.) politically and socially. The Confederation of Health Service Employees (C.O.H.S.E.) was again fully affiliated to the T.U.C., but never again attained primacy amongst the nursing unions and when on 3rd July 1974 a Shop Stewards Committee was formed of 12 members, 6 of them represented N.U.P.E. including the Chairman.

There was less optimism but the pattern of *The Glensider* under Linda still must cover hospital activities. A typical issue had the usual headings – welcome to newcomers and farewell to leavers, N.H.S. superannuation, Winners in Ward raffle, thanks to sponsored walker, Grand sale of Ward 9, Staff Social Club meeting and election of officers, don't forget firework display, lucky winner of food hamper, N.U.P.E. Grand night out, L Ward disco and dance and so on.

The futility of Area, District and Sector management, the turbulence which ensued post 1974 gave rise to little critical comment. Matters of contention were mainly avoided. The deterioration of manners was commented on. Violence also became a problem. Outbreaks at dances were reported at the Social Club in March 1979.

The proposal in 1980 to build an in-patient Forensic Unit met opposition with complaints from the public of a less than helpful attitude and by members of the hospital staff.

Administrative changes proposed in the Mental Health Act (1983) became operative (30th Sept 1983).

Staff became increasingly worried and suspicious. Through 1983 an atmosphere of secrecy pervaded the administration. In July Mrs Barbara Young, Chairman of Frenchay Health Authority issued a statement concerning the Hospital Advisory Service visit to Glenside. She described its tone as "perceptive, helpful and generally encouraging... there is much at Glenside of which we can be proud ... excellent foundations on which to build." She wrote of advice which might be taken to improve the less satisfactory aspects of Glenside but added that the Report was confidential and addressed to her. She would not make the contents public. It would be discussed collectively and individually with the members of the Unit Management Group and the District Officers would jointly prepare and implement a plan of action upon the reports findings. "Members of Glenside Hospital Staff may be reassured that we are looking towards taking positive steps in full consultation with individual groups of staff." There was no reassurance. No more was reported about these consultations in *The Glensider*.

The next communication reported from Mrs Young was a letter in November 1984 concerning the appointment of a District General manager and explaining his duties. "The District General Manager will take personal responsibility for advising the Health Authority and seeing that its policies are carried out." The job was in the Press, appointment would be in New Year. There would be discussions on future management structure of the Authority and the appointment of Hospital General Managers. The staff remained worried "about the long-term future of Glenside and the various rumours circulating." An open meeting for 6th December 1984 was called by the Management Group. There is no report on this meeting, nor if it took place at all but later in the month Mrs Young apologised for not visiting at Christmas because of pressure of work. In January 1985 she wrote that she was well aware of the interest and concern about "this important post" and hoped to make an announcement after the next meeting of the Health Authority on 21st January. After this meeting she wrote that "unfortunately it has not proved possible to make an appointment." Re-advertisement was immediate. Interviews to be held in Mid March. On April 4th she announced the appointment of Dr Paul Walker as District General Manager.

On 28th October 1985, Walter Mears a serving R.A.F. officer was appointed as Unit General Manager to Community Health, Mental Handicap and Mental Health each of which job had been advertised as a separate appointment. The Districts concerned raised continuing objections. Great exception was taken to this multiple appointment. Each of these three positions warranted the appointment of a separate officer. The triple appointment was made without consultation. Mrs Young later wrote an apologetic letter acknowledging her mistake and assuring the staff that there would be no recurrence of similar actions in the future. This letter was not published. It made no difference anyway. Squadron Leader Mears started his 3 year contract on 9th January 1986 and was stationed at Glenside.

The staff were unsettled. The following month David Cottingham, the Director of Nursing left the service. His farewell laudation described him as conscientious, dedicated and caring, epthithets with which his colleagues agreed. It made no mention of the circumstances of his retirement.

Mr Mears introduced a new sort of discipline. From 3rd March 1986 only designated staff were allowed in Admin Car Park and for the first time clamping was threatened. On September 18th it was further threatened publicly to "name & shame non-payers of private telephone calls." Apparently this threat was carried out, although not published in *The Glensider*. Forgiveness was published on 18th February 1987 for McDonald who has paid his telephone bill."

In April, the Editor Linda Gravesbecame Deputy Administrator. The Management shake up saw Alec Haslett transferred to Manor Park. His valedictory presentation from the Consultants was accompanied by a eulogy on the excellence of his character and of his contribution to Glenside.

The Wards were also disappearing one by one. On 2nd October 1987, it was reported that 11 patients from M Ward were discharged to Causeway House a hospital hostel with the statement; "M will no longer exist as a ward."

Linda's last edition of *The Glensider* was on 27th October 1988. Dave Paynes 1st edition was 3rd Oct 1988. He retained the time tested format whilst dispensing with much of the news.

His first major assignment was on 23rd December 1988. His "Thank you" to the retiring Squadron Leader "I assure you, you were not the boil you thought you were", did not meet with approval of all staff and was accorded an apology on 5th Jan '89.

Administration grew apace. New titles abounded. On 27 July'89 Kevin Hegarty was appointed Unit General Manager Glenside Community Services and on 15th October Bill Evans became Assistant General Manager. On 10th August 1988 Ward Managers and night co-ordinators were named "with effect from 13th August the following will commence their activities as Ward managers." The end of an era. The Ward Sister thus followed the Matron into oblivion. There was a price to be paid. On 12th October 1989 there was a full page advertisement for counselling "free sessions with an independent counsellor to all Frenchay staff."

By 1990 there is much less social news overall e.g. Ward parties and events trade union activities, retired staff meetings continue. The approach is colder than before although names are recorded in familiar style as on 22nd February 1990 when Senior Clinical Nurse specialists Helen, Sylvia, Kate were appointed. This intimate method of address was not however accorded to Male Nurse Edmond Luaynor, who was similarly promoted.

The closure of the Hospital ward by ward has not been recorded in detail, "A very difficult time for all, especially the patients" was foretold. It was planned that the United Bristol Hospitals should remove their patients in 1990 and accordingly Ward 9 (which opened as an undergraduate teaching unit in 1968) closed on 30th November 1990. Dr.Brown, Consultant Psychiatrist said good-bye; "Over the years the ward has played an active part in the life of Glenside and I regret that the need to consolidate Bristol and Weston services at Barrow Hospital has made its closure inevitable." In January 1991 the Ward reopened as a fast-flow rehab facility at the same time as Ward 14 reopened for the slower movers.

The issue of December 13th announced that an Information board detailing dates of ward closures and relocation of services would be displayed in the staff canteen "with effect from

Monday 17th December 1990." Information regarding vacancies for which staff could apply were also posted there and sent to the wards. Information pads were available on request.

December 20th announced the proposed date of closure of the Glenside site and an illustration of the Wards to be occupied in Manor Park. The first moves scheduled were the reopening of Wards 9 & 14 which were "successfully reopened" on 17th January. At this time H, K and L were closed. "The biggest reorganisation of Wards to take place in such a short space of time that I can remember" wrote the Editor who piloted the last *Glensider* to press on 31st January 1991. He mustered "A certain amount of sadness" for its passing.

It gave way to *Focus*, whose first number appeared on Friday 1st March 1991. It ran through 21 issues under various editors up to 8th January 1992. It carried little domestic news. It still welcomed 113 newcomers to the staff and bade farewell to 157 over the same period.

On 29th March the proposed opening of the Beaufort Unit (Manor Park) for the aged including the demented was announced for the following month. This Unit consisted of Bowood Day Unit, Blaise, Blenheim (25 beds) and Berkeley Wards with Badminton (20 beds) in the main building and Parkfield Day Hospital within Cossham Hospital (Kingswood). This manoeuvre was described as "part of continuing re-location of Frenchay Mental Health Service away from the main Victorian building at Glenside Hospital." On 8th April 1991, Ward 12 moved to Blenheim, on the 9th Ward 19 moved to Berkeley and on 10th B and Wickham Glen to Bowood. On 12th April it was announced that "the patients have settled in extremely well."

On 9th January 1992 Focus reported that a new unit was a building (cost £1,000,000) a 40 bedded unit in Blackberry Hill Hospital grounds (i.e. the re-named Manor Park) "to take the last of Frenchay's patients from the Victorian buildings of Glenside" for completion in September. "This is an integral part of the overall plan to provide an integrated community oriented mental health service" wrote Mr W.R.Evans, Manager of Frenchay Mental Health Directorate. "It will be safe accommodation in an attractive setting." [This was demolished in 2003.]

The local and national newspapers tell the story of terminal decline even more vividly but first the Trade Union situation must be clarified. At its foundation the Confederation of Health Service Employees (C.O.H.S.E.) became the official organisation of more than 40,000 workers within every branch of the Health service. It aimed to protect its members and to ensure that the new National Health Service should be established on firm and secure foundations. It achieved representation for almost 100% of the nursing staff of the Bristol Mental Hospital, (later Glenside Hospital).

Against the advice of the T.U.C., C.O.H.S.E. registered under the Heath Government's trade union legislation and thereby lost its immunity under the Bridlington agreement from canvassing within the hospital by other Trade Unions. This allowed the National Union of Public Employees (N.U.P.E.) to canvas for members and to establish a Glenside Hospital branch in 1972. Thereafter the representation of the nursing staff was split between these two unions, together with the Royal College of Nursing (R.C.N.) and a small number represented by the Transport and General Workers Union (T.G.W.U.). N.U.P.E, the new comer, became the most active.

The Front Office, the administrative staff, kept a newspaper cuttings book relating to the hospital from February 1954 to August 1992, mainly local papers, the *Western Daily Press* (W.D.P.) and the Evening Post (E.P). All are preserved in the Glenside Hospital Museum. Up to 1973 no industrial dispute is reported.
The Health Service re-organisation of 1974 led to management of Glenside Hospital being taken over by Frenchay General Hospital, the management of which hospital was seen by Glenside staff as being ignorant of the problems of the mental hospital and interested mainly in cutting costs by reducing services. The near chaos that surrounded the re-organisation

produced instability and uncertainty. In the run up to the transfer of power to District Management, the staff lost confidence in the management and was unhappy, fearful and unsettled. In November the staff voted no confidence in the future. Within a few months, 200 nurses in Western hospitals were working to rule, maintenance departments withdrew good will from management and the laundry was again in chaos. The unsettled state continued so that in September and again in November, Jerry Walker, the local M.P. sought an enquiry into Glenside staffing. This was claimed in *The Glensider* to be the first ever. A "Hospital staff Crisis" headline in the Evening Post on July 4th the same year confirmed that the dispute was on-going.

Dispute followed dispute. There were 14 unions represented on the hospital staff. The nurses were the largest group of employees. They spread their wings and for the first time since 1891, on 12th & 13th March 1974, two weeks before the dismissal of the Hospital Management Committee N.U.P.E. took industrial action, short of outright withdrawal of labour. Lengthy discussions absorbed much valuable nursing time to reach an agreement on the second day of the dispute. Peace did not last long. The unhappy atmosphere bubbled on and reached breaking point the following month in April 1974.

Again withdrawal of labour was not complete but on this occasion C.O.H.S.E. joined forces with N.U.P.E. The R.C.N. did not take part. Once more an agreement was cobbled together in a few days and an uneasy peace prevailed. A dispute over nursing insistence that the hospital did not have the facilities to admit a dangerous patient, soured inter-professional relations culminating in the local MP publicly asking for an enquiry into the level of nursing staff in the hospital. The pot boiled over in October 1975 when there was a stand taken by N.U.P.E., against the admission of a capital patient leading to a headline in the Daily Express "Union forces Court to jail sick killer, Mr Justice, Shop Steward." Almost 6 months later (March 1976) a neighbouring hospital accepted the patient but months of bitterness and recrimination continued after the settlement of this dispute. Union refusal to admit violent patients was a recurring theme but opposition to the building of a specialised forensic unit persisted. In June 1983, the Daily Mail reported that the Health Unions were in danger of being held in contempt of Court for refusal to admit but on September 9th a Judge was forced to release a woman because no hospital vacancy could be found for her.

Often more than one dispute was going on simultaneously. These took an inordinate amount of time even when the Union was carrying out one of its fundamental duties – the protection of jobs and wages.

Representation of management views were often presented by Officers with little authority and of comparatively junior standing often supported too late by their seniors who were far removed from the work place where the dispute had arisen. During one such dispute on 12th and 13th March 1976 the Hospital Divisional Officer and a Nursing Officer, supported by their weak Sector Administrator faced strong and aggressive Union Stewards. Settlement was delayed until the second day of negotiations when higher nursing management in the person of the Area Nursing Officer joined the fray and an agreement was reached.

INDUSTRIAL ACTION BY MEMBERS OF N.U.P.E. ON 12TH & 13TH MARCH,1976.

On Thursday, 11th March, 1976, Mr. Cottongham (Divisional Nursing Officer) and Mr Haslett (Sector Administrator) were called to a meeting of the N.U.P.E. Executive Committee and were informed that with effect from 7a.m. on Friday 12th, March all nursing staff members of N.U.P.E. would be instructed to refrain from:

1.	Changing shifts;	)
2.	Changing days off;	)See copy attached of
3.	Altering previously agreed leave;	)document circulated
4.	Carrying out unpaid duties in a higher grade;	)to ALL NURSING
5.	Taking time off in lieu or working overtime.	)MEMBERS (N.U.P.E.)

The reason given for this was that the union felt that there was a need for an increase in the number of trained staff on the wards at Glenside and yet at the same time the student and pupil nurses who were shortly expecting their final examination results were not being offered substantive posts as Staff Nurses or S.E.N.'s. An urgent meeting was requested with Mrs.E.Y.Atkinson District Nursing Officer and via her, Mr.R.Bennett, Area Nursing Officer.

Following this meeting a meeting was arranged for 11.30 on Friday morning which was attended by the following:

Mrs .Y.Atkinson, District Nursing Officer
Mr.P.May, Associate District Administrator
Mr.D.Cottingham, Divisional Nursing Officer
Mr.C.A.Haslett, Sector Administrator
Mr.R.McLellan, Nursing Officer
Mr.J.McAvinney)
Mr.J.Goold) Representative of N.U.P.E.
Mr.R.Punter) Stewards
(Mr.R.Bennett, Area Nursing Officer was unable to be present).

At this meeting it was explained that no additional monies were available within the District to fund additional trained posts within the Sector and as the number of trained staff currently employed was in excess of the funded establishment it was not possible to offer any of the students or pupil nurses who would shortly be qualifying, trained posts within Glenside. However, following lengthy discussions it was agreed to continue the meeting in the afternoon during which time the following were present:

Mr.Cottingham
Mr. Haslett
Mr.McLellan
Mr. McAvinney
Mr. Goold

And for part of the time Mr.C.Hay, District Personnel Officer.

Consideration was given to a number of suggestions as to ways in which posts could be found for these student and pupil nurses concerned, and it was eventually agreed that consideration should be given to the issuing to student nurses who applied for Staff Nurse posts and who are successful in passing their final examination and who would normally have received a month's notice with effect from 1st April, 1976, of limited term contracts as staff nurse for a period of two months from the date of their individual E.N.C.

Registration (approx.1st April, 1976) with an agreement that, if they still had not been successful in obtaining either further training or a substantive post elsewhere, they would be given a further similar contract for another two months, after which their employment at Glenside would be terminated without further notice. In this way it was hoped that the majority of the students who would receive their results at the end of March would be given a "breathing space" in which to find further employment.

On the basis of this offer the N.U.P.E. representative agreed to call a meeting of their Executive Committee on Friday evening. This was held and the union agreed to suspend industrial action for night shift commencing on Friday, 11th March, pending a further meeting with the Area Nursing Officer arranged for 10.00a.m. Saturday morning, 13th March, 1976.

On Saturday, 13th March at 10a.m. a further meeting was held at which the following were present:

Mr.R.Bennett, Area Nursing Officer
Mrs.Y.Atkinson, District Nursing Officer
Mr.D.Cottingham, Divisional Nursing Officer
Mr.R.McLellan, Nursing Officer
Miss. S.Hook, Senior Nursing Officer (Personnel)
Mr. C.A.Haslett, Sector Administrator
Mr.C.Hay, District Personnel Officer

Mr.J.McAvinney)
Mr.R.Punter   )
Mr.A.Kettle   )
Mr.G.Jenkins   )   N.U.P.E Stewards
Mrs.K.Stone   )
Mr.R.Honeywell   )
Mr.A.Boadu   )
Mr.B.English   )

At this meeting Mr.Bennett confirmed that no funds for additional trained nursing staff posts would be available to Avon Area in the coming financial year and that any posts for trained staff at Glenside over and above the existing establishment would have to be funded from within the existing nursing staff budget.

Following further lengthy discussions it was agree:

1. That limited term contracts on the lines outlined above should be issued to those student nurses who wish to take advantage of them and who receive confirmation of their success in their final examinations at the end of March;

2. That similar contracts be issued to those pupil nurses who wish to take advantage of them and who receive confirmation of their success at the end of May 1976;

3. That the situation be reviewed in June 1976 prior to and on receipt of the results of the next finalists (student and pupils) with a view to making similar arrangements for those students and pupils;

4. That the funding of these limited term contracts which would further increase the number of trained staff in post should be found by;
    a. having fewer learners in post than the fund establishment
    b. allowing the natural wastage of untrained staff over the year to reduce the overall number of nurses in post; the <u>funded</u> establishment of 391.6 remaining unaltered[e.g. 10 Nursing Assistants 'wasted' (at current salary mean of scale) = 10 x £ 20,000 which equates to approx 7.5 trained staff (taking mean of Staff Nurse and S.E.N. scales)] and (c)   if necessary budget underspendings within the Sector an be re-deployed on a non-recurring basis by agreement with the appropriate heads of department and the S.M.T.;

5. That, as a matter of policy, nursing staff who retire should not be re-employed on a part-time, year to year, basis and that existing staff employed on this basis should not be renewed when their present contracts fall due for review;

6. That current District policy regarding the continuing employment of staff who have attained pensionable age be positively followed;

7. That current N.H.S. policy regarding the employment of nursing staff over 60 be reaffirmed. The individual cases of staff over 60 years who have achieved their maximum pension rights should be critically examined;

8. That the numbers of trained staff be maintained at the present level subject to review in relation to the needs of patient care by the District Nursing Officer as a matter of urgency.

This offer was accepted by the N.U.P.E. Executive Committee who consequently decided to end the industrial action immediately

The Seventies, the years of re-organisation start with an explosion of unhappiness and dissatisfaction. The Evening Post of June 8th 1973 headlined "Laundry Staff Walk out at Glenside." From there on it is nearly all downhill. Ninety-three (93) cuttings followed the laundry dispute. Eight (8) relate to industrial unrest in that department, six (6) to similar action by the Nursing staff, four (4) to general staff courses, three (3) to kitchen workers and one each to drivers and machine operators. The quarrels were related to pay and conditions of service related to the present and future plans for the hospital.

Administrative proposals to use Ham Green Hospital as an admission site were seen by the staff as a *fait accompli*: "Row looms over ward switch plan – EP 9th July 1976. The Avon

Area Health Authority met the staff who were protesting against what they saw as a Weston-Super-Mare/Bristol merger.

The kitchen staff (NUPE and COHSE) walked out on 16th/17th November 1979 over a check of kitchen stock books. Four months later 80 cleaners, cooks, laundry workers and porters, mainly T.G.W.U. members, walked out because of the sacking of one of their members.

So it went on month after month with only one happy note by James Belsey in the Evening Post on 2nd December 1981, reporting celebration dinner of the 25th Anniversary of the Industrial Therapy Organisation: "Amazing success, incredulous world."

The number of industrial disputes, go-slows and stoppages reported gave way to disciplinary charges mostly against nurses. On 20th December 1982 the Post reported that 7 nurses were under suspension and next day that they were sacked. A special visit of the Health Advisory Service in September '83 reported low staff morale and manpower shortages. Within a week a nurse was cleared of attacking a man and a few days later a Charge Nurse and a female nursing auxiliary were suspended for stealing. There were claims of misbehaviour by 7 other nurses and a final warning was given to an auxiliary nurse for striking a patient. Within a year, 11 staff had been suspended but to cap it all this, the Nursing Officer was sent home on full pay (31st October 1983) as was the Chairman of the Glenside branch of N.U.P.E. "for exceeding Union powers." The Chairman did not return; the Nursing Officer did on 17th November but he left in July 1986.

On 4th December 1985, a House of Commons Select Committee was set up to enquire into the management of the Frenchay Health District by Mrs Barbara Young, Chairman and Dr Paul Walker Chief Executive.

As related before, R.A.F. Wing Commander W. Mears was appointed Unit General Manager on 27th November 1985. The circumstances of the appointment did not engender confidence. He had no experience of hospital management.

Unrest continued. Funding for staff was inadequate as it was for community projects. The prospect of the sack was never far away. Industrial Action was always pending. On 29th January 1988 the *Post* reported that "for the first time", the Nurses had voted for strike. The *Bristol Observer* (19/02/88) spoke of "Slave labour" YTS trainees in charge of Wards. The Nurses picketed the hospital for 1 day on 25th February 1988 and on March 3rd, the *Evening Post* reported "Strikers on the March." They got a pay rise but the dispute continued.

In May 1988 a new Chief Executive Mrs Ann Lloyd was appointed to the Frenchay District.

Headlines continued to be dramatic: "Scandal of West's Asylums" (E.P. 28/06/88) and the pay dispute continued. Nurses considered that they had been cheated and went on strike on 11th November and continued so, until they called a truce on 16th December. They felt angry because their pay was lower than other districts, angry because they regarded the highly paid Agency Nurses as strike breakers and angry because they felt degraded (E.P. 22/11/88). Nevertheless, they called a pay truce on 16th December 1988.

Fury broke out again in February 1989 when Glenside and Manor Park Hospital were amalgamated and it was announced that Glenside would close "within the year." To add painful uncertainty to uncertainty it didn't and it was announced that the closure would take place in July 1991 (*Evening Post* 24th January 1991). Again this did not occur and staff members were not assured by the absence of plans for staff "Axe to fall on 70 hospital jobs" announced the *Evening Post* on October 24th 1991.

After this only three further clips remain.

The *Evening Post* reported on 29th November 1991 that there were mice and cockroaches in the kitchen of Glenside. Nobody was surprised.

On August 8th 1992, the same newspaper reported that on the following day Mrs Bottomley the Secretary of State for Health "will unveil a plaque to commemorate the opening of the new Health College on Blackberry Hill", to cope with more than 1000 students, at a cost of £2,000,000. She was officially opening the Avon College of Health, later the Avon and Gloucester College of Health and now the Faculty of Health and Social Care of the University of the West of England.

The Thatcher revolution saw a radical reduction of union powers. Neither C.O.H.S.E nor N.U.P.E. now survive independently. They each tried in their own way to safeguard staff and patient rights against often ill-informed administrations whom they saw, as did many others as motivated by financial and political rather than by social and medical motives. They were not always wrong. On 1st July 1993, the three existing independent Trade Unions, the Confederation of Health Service Employees, (C.O.H.S.E), the National and Local Government Officers (N.A.L.G.O.) and the National Union of Public Employees (N.U.P.E.) joined to form one Union U.N.I.S.O.N now the single largest Trade Union in Great Britain.

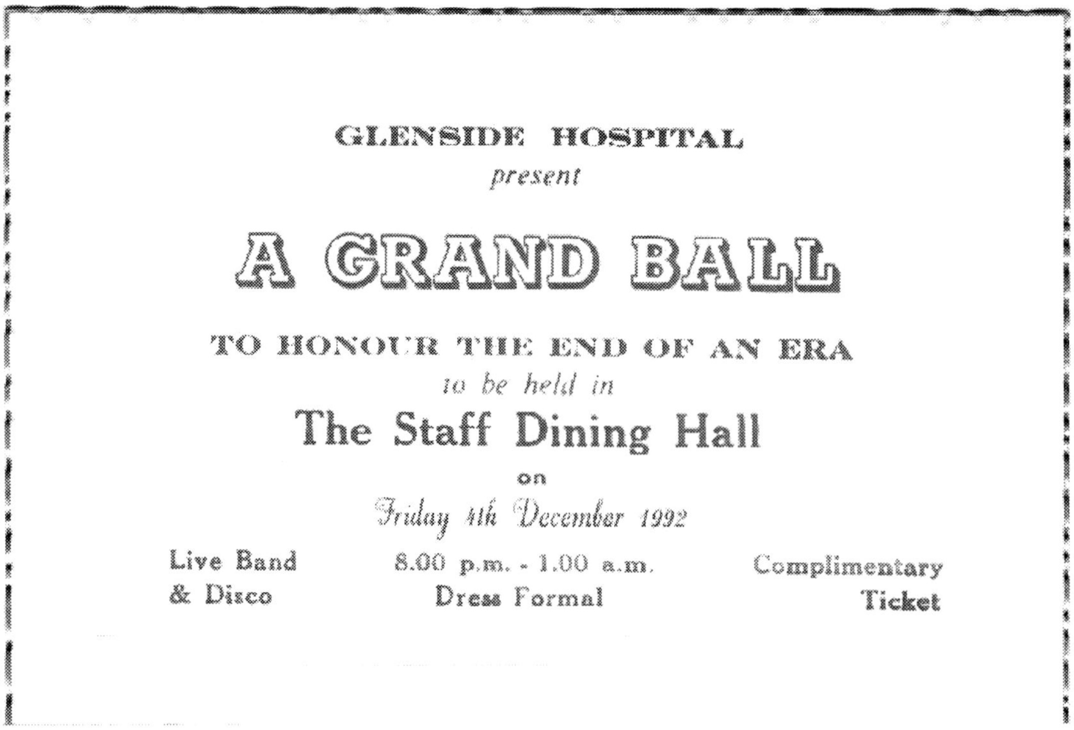

GLENSIDE HOSPITAL

present

A GRAND BALL

TO HONOUR THE END OF AN ERA

to be held in

The Staff Dining Hall

on

Friday 4th December 1992

Live Band   8.00 p.m. - 1.00 a.m.   Complimentary
& Disco   Dress Formal   Ticket

Figure 68 The Closing Ball

The Parallel Story: Blackberry Hill Hospital

Stapleton Prison 1779 ▶ Ordinance Store ▶ Stapleton Workhouse ▶ Stapleton Public Assistance Institution (PAI) 1918 ▶ Stapleton Hospital 1948 ▶ Manor Park Hospital ▶ Blackberry Hill Hospital (1992)

Blackberry Hill Hospital has had a chequered history. Its early days up to 1837 are recorded by Dorothy Vinter in *Transactions of the Bristol & Gloucestershire Archaeological Society* Vol. 75, 1950. A short booklet entitled *A History of Manor Park Hospital; 150 years of Caring 1832 – 1982* written by Mrs Jean Nelson was published and circulated privately in 1982, and briefly deals with the workhouse and hospital years.

The prison accommodation in Bristol was insufficient to accommodate prisoners of war taken as the result of the revolution of the American colonies in 1775 and of the war with France and Spain in 1778 and 1779. A new prison was built at Stapleton on the site of the present Blackberry Hill Hospital and opened for the reception of prisoners in 1779 when 150 convicts were transferred from the prison at Redcliffe Back (Bristol). During the next three years more than 2,000 Spanish prisoners were housed there but it was mainly the French who suffered its harsh regime when war broke out again in 1793, after 10 years of peace.

Whilst used as a prison, conditions were generally poor and subject to gross overcrowding. In 1798 when the population of the prison was 2,000 there was a request for admission of 700 Frenchmen allied to the Irish in the rebellion of that year. A new building had to be provided in 1800. At the time of the French Revolution things got so bad that Mr Batchelor a deputy Governor of St Peter's Hospital and Mr Andrews, a Quaker, having visited the prison described how the prisoners were nearly naked, without shoes or stockings and walking in the courtyard 4 inches deep in mud. It was said that the prisoners themselves were partly to blame because of their gambling and selling their clothes to buy food and tobacco. Four hundred and fifty of them had no clothes at all and such a large number required help that at the personal behest of the King, the Government took responsibility for prison clothing because "His Majesty could no longer continue to consider the men as French prisoners but as destitute fellow creatures." (Rosser and Moore Pamphlet Bristol Central Library).

Conditions continued to be bad. In November and December 1800, 200 deaths were recorded. In 1805, 220 cases of Typhus were reported; in 1807 pulmonary tuberculosis was rife and 80 patients had pneumonia; there was an outbreak of smallpox in March 1809. Many deaths took place from duels which occurred about once weekly. During epidemics the bodies were placed in piles, head to foot and three groups were buried together. During excavations for hospital developments skeletons have been found thus positioned.

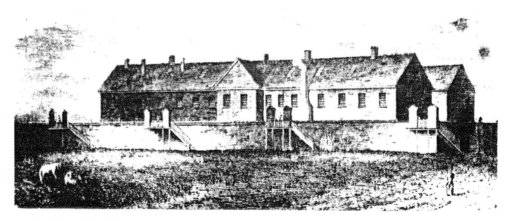

Figure 69 Stapleton Prison

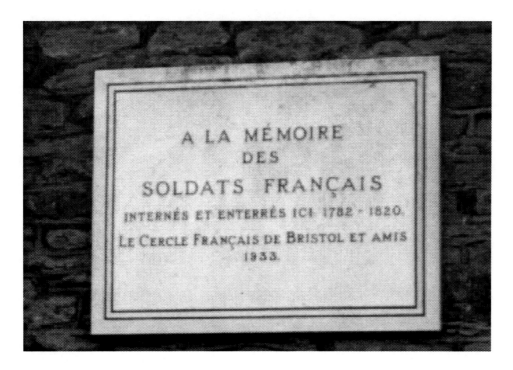

Figure 70 Memorial Plaque

Their ordeals are commemorated by a plaque erected by the Cercle Francais de Bristol in memory of the interred and the interned, who were victims of the war until the Treaty of Paris in 1814.

The Treaty of Paris brought the release of 2,000 prisoners. Stapleton was never again used as a prison. It became an Ordnance Store until the cholera epidemic of 1832 when part was rented by the Incorporation of the Poor to relieve the extreme overcrowding at St Peter's. The following year it was purchased by this body and used as a workhouse, always an important element in the care of pauper lunatics. It was a frequent resting-place for the indigent mentally ill who were not acceptable in the community.

In 1854 it was suggested as a lunatic asylum, which proposition was refused by the Incorporation of the Poor. Later in a gesture of desperation they offered it for this use but this was firmly rejected by the Commissioners in Lunacy.

Between 1861 and 1865 new buildings were erected on the site, of which E Block is left standing. In 1918 the workhouse came under the Board of Guardians and was later known as Stapleton Public Assistance Institution (PAI). It was incorporated in the National Health Service in July 1948 as Stapleton Hospital.

Early on an administrative problem arose from the change of status. The main groups of patients in the Institution were those detained under Sections 24, 25 and 20 of the Lunacy Act 1890 and those detained under the Mental Deficiency Acts 1913 and 1927. The detention of these categories of patients imposed the statutory requirement that the hospital should have a Medical Superintendent. This fact had apparently not been appreciated by the legislators so in 1949 it was somewhat of a panic measure that the Medical Superintendent of the Bristol Mental Hospital was asked to undertake this responsibility. In spite of the impracticality of this, an immediate solution was urgent and there was no obvious alternative. The title was nominally accepted by the Medical Superintendent of the Mental Hospital and was carried out in an "acting" capacity by the physician in charge of Fishponds Hospital.

The general medical administration of the Stapleton General Hospital devolved upon Dr W. Broadfoot who came from Frenchay Hospital as Medical Superintendent. Douglas Pearson erstwhile Master of the Institution became the Hospital Secretary and his wife, the Matron. Dr S. S. Datta was the only medical officer already in post and he acted mainly as a G.P. to the patients. Unlike the Mental Hospital there were no rules requiring periodical clinical examination of inmates and so there were no comprehensive medical records.

The South Western Regional Hospital Board requested a medical and psychiatric assessment of the inmates. I undertook a rapid superficial patient review in 1947 and followed this with a detailed survey of the hospital population, in August 1949.

The major categories of patients in the hospital were:
1. Patients ascertained under the Mental Deficiency Acts 1913 and 1927 of whom there were 76 female and 73 male patients (149). The hospital was licensed for the care of 200 such patients.
2. Three hundred and fifty five 'certified' patients (233 female, 122 male), all ambulant and detained under Secs 24 and 25 of the Lunacy Act 1890, These were described in 4 categories and recommendations made for each category.
3. Uncertified patients who were ambulant and confined to various wards throughout the hospital. There were 97 in this category (30 men and 67 women). These were classified into 6 categories and recommendations made in each case. The legality of the detention of many of these was doubtful.
4. Sick Hospital – 242 patients (176 female and 66 male)
5. Observation Wards (Secs 20, 21, 21A of the Lunacy Act) 8 male, 12 female.

STAPLETON HOSPITAL

A detailed survey of the patients was begun early in March 1949 and was completed last week.
The major categories of patients in hospital are:
  I. Mental defectives ascertained as such, of which there are 157 (on 20.8.49). None of those seen except 11 who were in the Sick Blocks at the time of the survey.
 II. Uncertified patients who were ambulant and confined in various wards throughout the hospital. I have listed these under (a) Those who are possibly suitable for home or local authority; (b) those who are suitable for mental hospital treatment; (c) those who are bedridden; (d) those whom admission to Bristol Mental Hospital might benefit; (e) those not considered psychotic, whom it is proposed to ask the Mental Deficiency Authorities to see, and (f) those who are frail and ambulant. I have also made a list of those who are definitely not willing to remain in hospital. As will be seen by the note accompanying this list, the legality of the detention of many more of these is doubtful.
III. Certified patients ambulant at the time of survey. These total 330; 111 males and 219 females. (A further 30 certified patients are dealt with under the heading of Sick Hospital). I have listed these patients under the following headings: (a) those suitable for mental hospital treatment; (b) those whom admission to Bristol Mental Hospital might benefit; (c) those suitable for home or local authority, and (d) those considered psychotic, and whom it is proposed to ask the Mental Deficiency Authorities to see.
 IV. Sick Hospital. I have listed these under; Ascertained Mentally Defectives; Section 24; and Uncertified, and the proposed method of dealing with each case is dealt with individually in these lists.
I have also listed Age Groups of patients, from a point of view of interest.

Due to the length of time taken over the survey there will be some minor inaccuracies due to discharges or death, but the total picture will be fairly accurate.

The outstanding feature of the survey is the large number of patients certified under the Lunacy Acts whom I consider to be mentally defective. There is little doubt that the majority of these patients are so, but here again there may be some inaccuracies as the decision was made as a result of one psychiatric interview, and the amount of subsidiary information available was small.

FISHPONDS

The Mental Hospital at Fishponds was also surveyed during this period. I append a list of patients who might possibly be dealt with elsewhere, and a list of patients who may benefit by leucotomy. The age groupings and percentages of each group have also been worked out.

REGIONAL BOARD CLASSIFICATIONS

The classification requested by the Regional Board has been carried out in both hospitals. I have not found these classifications useful, and in the case of the Mental Hospital there were several who could not be classified under the 4 headings given.

In Stapleton the numbers of mentally defective are drawn from those certified under the Lunacy Acts and considered mentally defective, certified under the Mental Deficiency Acts.

A detailed report and recommendations were made for the care of the aged bed-fast patients, many of them mentally intact. The speciality of geriatrics was currently being rediscovered. I visited many centres and derived major help and guidance from Dr Marjory Warren of the West Middlesex County Hospital, Isleworth following which an outline plan was presented to the H.M.C. of Stapleton Hospital including recommendations regarding staff and equipment. The report was, accepted and later Dr William Hughes the first Consultant Geriatrician in Bristol was appointed with the brief to establish a centre at Stapleton Hospital for the investigation and treatment of patients suffering from diseases of old age.

LONG-STAY UNIT. STAPLETON

On Thursday, 15th September 1949, I called on Dr. Marjorie Warren, of the West Middlesex County Hospital, Isleworth, to discuss the question of the establishment of a long-stay hospital.

She considers (and I agree) that the buying of equipment for such a hospital is largely a waste if the staffing has not first been established. She considers that such staffing should form part of the formation of such a unit.

Staffing:
    The Following categories are essential:
        1) Doctors
        2) Physiotherapists
        3) Occupational Therapists
        4) Almoners

Doctors: Dr Warren's present unit has about 180 beds, for which she has 3 doctors – herself, and 2 House Officers. The establishment for which she hopes for is 5, adding a Senior Officer and a Registrar to her present establishment. On the basis of her present number of doctors, 4 medical men would be necessary in Stapleton, a Consultant, a Senior Hospital Officer, and 2 House Officers. The salary ranges of these would be from £3,700 a year to £5,400 a year.

Physiotherapists: To start with 1 Physiotherapist, who would, of course, be in sole charge, and the salary range of such a person would be £350 to £400 a year.

Occupational Therapists: To start with 1 single-handed Occupation Therapist, salary range £ 400 to £ 450 a year.

<u>Almoners</u>: To start with 1 senior single-handed Almoner, salary range £380 to £455 a year.

Thus the total salaries for the initial staff would be somewhere in the range of £4,830 to £6,715 a year. It is emphasised that if this department is developed further staff would undoubtedly be required.

The equipping of these departments is the next consideration. It should come under the heading of equipment, but I have put it down separately.

<u>Medical Officers</u>: 1 office for medical officers, with office equipment. Roughly £250.

<u>Physiotherapy Department</u>: I have had an estimate from Stanley Cox Ltd. Who have equipped several complete departments recently, such as Longthorn Hospital, Leytonstone, Essex, and they give the approximate cost for such a department as from £550 to £600. This will include such things as short wave unit and various forms of gymnastic equipment, combined electronic tables, etc.

<u>Occupational Therapy</u>: The cost of equipment and materials to start such a department would be about £350. I arrived at this figure in consultation with our Supplies Officer.

<u>Almoner</u>: The equipping of an Almoner's office would initially cost about £220.

Thus, the equipping of these departments would come to approximately £1,420.00

I discussed individual equipment with Dr.Warren, and the proportion of the various items of equipment which would be required for our department. The following are the most important items:

1)	Guthrie Smith Sling. 1 complete (Stanley Cox Ltd.)	£47	19	9
2)	Ward Model Suspension Apparatus.(Stanley Cox Ltd.) 2 @ £20	40	-	-
3)	Balken Beams (Stanley Cox Ltd.). 6 @ £3/17/6	23	5	-
4)	Portable Bed Exercise Apparatus. (Stanley Cox Ltd.) 4 @ £15/15/-	63	-	-
5)	Bed Cradles (1 to 5). 33 @ approx. 17/-	28	1	-
6)	Lifting Poles (1 to 2). 120 @ £2/1/6	249	-	-
7)	Walking Machines (1 per floor). 3 @ £14/14/-	44	2	-
8)	Wheel Chairs (1 to 5):			
	35 Edinburgh Type (Willen Bros.) @ £15	525	-	-
	15 Stairchair Type (Willen Bros.) @ £9/8/6	141	7	6
9)	High Stools (1 to 15):			
	Wheel Type. 8 @ approx £14	112	-	-
	Chair Type. 8 @ approx £9/11/3	76	10	-
10)	Sanitary Chairs (wheel-chair stools): (1 per floor). 3 @ £17	51	-	-
11)	Oxygen Equipment: 3 sets @ approx. £12	36	-	-
12)	Fowlers Beds: 6 @ £22	132.	-.	-.
13)	Miscellaneous equipment: walking sticks with rubber ferrules, crutches, lead shot, webbing, sand bags, holding bars, additional springs: approximately	100	-	-
		£ 1,699	5s	3d

Thus, the total amount of the items listed, including salaries, is from £7,672 to £9,557. This does not include such items, which I consider desirable, as new floor coverings (highly polished floors are most undesirable in the treatment of old people), the painting of beds so as to get rid of the maze of black in the wards, and such other theatre and specialised orthopaedic equipment as will undoubtedly be necessary if the hospital becomes established.

I would point out that the establishment of such a unit is comparable to the establishment of a surgical unit, and should be treated accordingly.

Further expenses will undoubtedly arise, and a further amount for immediate contingency should be allowed.

Continuing consultant psychiatric advice was invited for the Observation Wards which received and dealt with patients admitted under Sec. 20 of the Lunacy Act. Under this section, Relieving Officers and Police Officers had the right and the duty to admit for a period of 3 days observation, patients suffering from symptoms of mental illness. The Relieving Officers [RO] became Duly Authorised Officers [DAO] in 1948. Prior to this date they used their powers as RO's under the Poor Laws Institution Order (1913) to order the Master of the workhouse to admit a wide range of cases often social rather than psychiatric. They had admission access to many different locations. Under their new title these same persons continued to be called on by general practitioners and by others to deal with the same problems. Subject to unchanged pressures after July 1948, the DAO now could obtain admission only under Sec. 20 of the Lunacy Act, i.e.: a 3 day order. The numbers of patients thus dealt with increased. In 1947 the last full year before the N.H.S. there were 212 admissions on 3-Day Orders to the Observation Wards of Stapleton Institution. Three-quarters of these were later certified and admitted to the Bristol Mental Hospital (B.M.H.).

After 1948 the wards continued to be designated for the purpose of Sec. 20 and 21 of the Lunacy Act. In 1954 a self-contained unit replaced the old Observation Wards. This consisted of contiguously situated wards containing 9 male and 12 female beds for Sec. 20 – 21 patients and an annexe of 18 female beds to deal with cases outside the Lunacy and Mental Treatment Acts. This unit of 39 beds (30 female, 9 male) was well furnished and equipped. It had its own part-time Medical Officer, Dr P. E. Early and was under the supervision of a doubly trained departmental nursing sister Miss M. Giles supported by trained psychiatric nursing staff. Admissions rapidly increased, reaching 620 in 1956. In the impending shadow of the Mental Health Act 1959 the numbers dwindled to 516 in 1957, 436 in 1958, 405 in 1959 and 330 in 1960.

In October 1961 the ward was handed over to Dr Michael Nicholas, Consultant Psychogeratrician with the intention of providing a tripartite assessment unit for the elderly confused patient with access to the psychiatric, geriatric and local authority services. Thus ended, for the time being, the long-standing and often-reluctant relationship between the workhouse and the asylum.

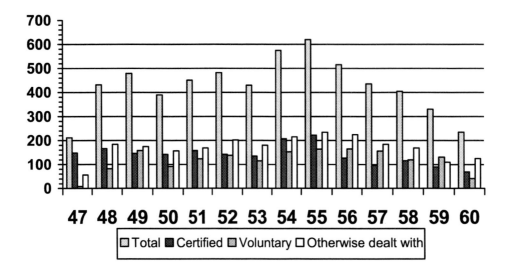

Figure 71 Admissions to Observation Ward 1947 - 1960

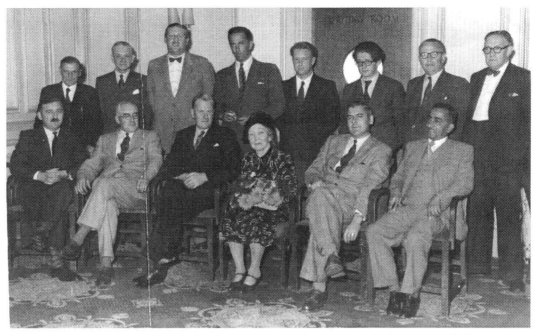

Mr A.J.Hewlett (DAO); Mr A.Saunders (DAO); Dr.K.C.P.Smith(Psych.Registrar); Dr Greville Elliott(GP); →
Dr.S.Pugmire (MO), Dr.A.McLennon (MO), Mr W.G.Morris (DAO), Mr A.H. Jordon (DAO).
Dr.D.F.Early, Dr.J.Moreton Evans (GP), Mr Frank Morton (Chief Mental Health Services), →
Mrs Edith Robinson White JP, Dr.W.L.Broadfoot (Medical Superintendent); Dr.S.Datta (Senior Medical Officer)

Figure 72 Observation Ward 14 Sept 1952

In its day, the Observation Ward fulfilled major medical, medico-legal and social roles. Patients were admitted by the D.A.O. usually at the request of a general practitioner. A magistrate visited thrice weekly with a doctor of his or her choosing. Mrs Edith Robinson-White J.P. gave outstanding service and became very knowledgeable and skilful in dealing with psychiatric problems.

However, the Councillors of 1858 had their belated way when in 1994/95 the remnant of patients from Glenside Hospital were transferred to psychiatric units on the site of Stapleton P.A.I. which now after many changes of name had metamorphosed into Blackberry Hill Hospital. The successors of eighteen-sixty-one's lunatics thereby ultimately inherited the work-house leaving to the Faculty of Health and Social Care of the University of the West of England, the Lunatic Pauper Palace (*Bristol Mercury* Oct 10th 1856), the palace with pleasure grounds (*Bristol Gazette* October 1855). The fortunate recipients of higher education in the nineteen nineties will hopefully be more appreciative of their surroundings than the lunatics of 1855 who according to the Corporation of the time did not require a fine place to reside in. And so this beautiful estate, this "princely domain" will happily continue in the service of the ill, for whom it was so hard won nearly a century and a half ago.

Illustration Sources and acknowledgements

All B&W images are from the Glenside Hospital Museum Collection.

Colour plates of Paintings of Stanley Spencer are reproductions of his work in the Sandham Memorial Chapel. Reproduced with permission © Estate of Stanley Spencer 2003, All Rights Reserved DACS. They are published from the National Trust Photographic Library, courtesy of National Trust, photographed by: J. Whitaker (Sorting the laundry) and Roy Fox (Bedmaking, Ablutions, Scrubbing the Floor, Moving Kitbags, Frostbite and Filling Tea Urns).

Glenside Hospital Museum
U.W.E. Glenside Campus
Stapleton
Bristol BS16 1DD

Open
Wednesdays and Saturdays
10am – 12.30pm

Buses: 5 stops outside
        48/49 pass through Fishponds
        4 passes through Stapleton to Frenchay

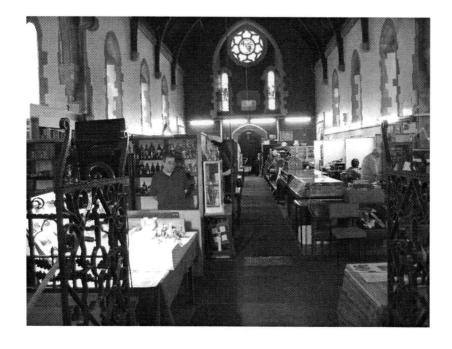

Index